a–z of learning disability

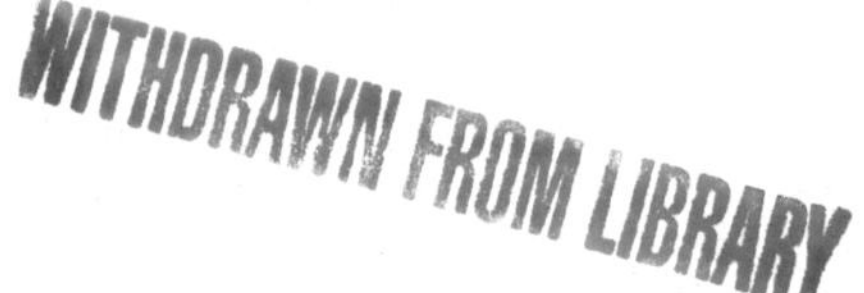

## Professional Keywords series

Every field of practice has its own methods, terminology, conceptual debates and landmark publications. The *Professional Keywords* series expertly structures this material into easy-reference A to Z format. Focusing on the ideas and themes that shape the field, these books are designed both to guide the student reader and to refresh practitioners' thinking and understanding.

**Available now**

Mark Doel and Timothy B. Kelly: *A–Z of Groups & Groupwork*
David Garnett: *A–Z of Housing*
Jon Glasby and Helen Dickinson: *A–Z of Interagency Working*
Richard Hugman: *A–Z of Professional Ethics*
Divya Jindal-Snape: *A–Z of Transitions*
Glenn Laverack: *A–Z of Health Promotion*
Glenn Laverack: *A–Z of Public Health*
Jeffrey Longhofer: *A–Z of Psychodynamic Practice*
Neil McKeganey: *A–Z of Addiction and Substance Misuse*
Steve Nolan and Margaret Holloway: *A–Z of Spirituality*
Angela Olsen, Andrea Pepe and Dan Redfearn: *A–Z of Learning Disability*
Marian Roberts: *A–Z of Mediation*
Fiona Timmins: *A–Z of Reflective Practice*
David Wilkins, David Shemmings and Yvonne Shemmings: *A–Z of Attachment*

a–z of

# learning disability

Angela Olsen, Andrea Pepe
& Dan Redfearn

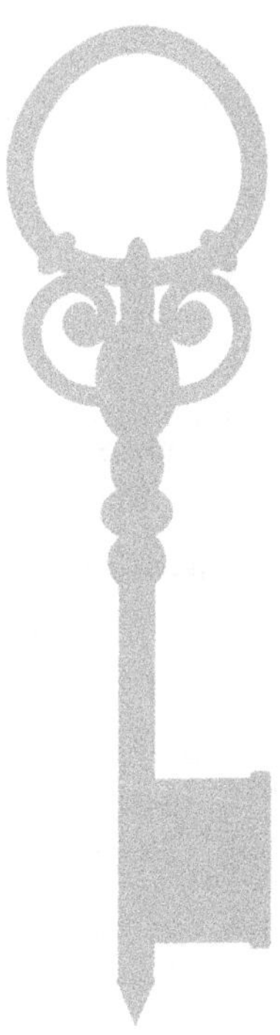

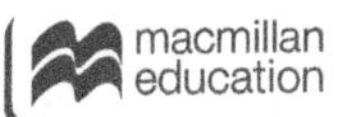


palgrave

First published 2017 by
PALGRAVE

Palgrave in the UK is an imprint of Macmillan Publishers Limited, registered in England, company number 785998, of 4 Crinan Street, London, N1 9XW.

Palgrave Macmillan in the US is a division of St Martin's Press LLC, 175 Fifth Avenue, New York, NY 10010.

Palgrave is a global imprint of the above companies and is represented throughout the world.



ISBN 978–1–137–47120–8 paperback

This book is printed on paper suitable for recycling and made from fully managed and sustained forest sources. Logging, pulping and manufacturing processes are expected to conform to the environmental regulations of the country of origin.

A catalogue record for this book is available from the British Library.

A catalog record for this book is available from the Library of Congress.

# contents

# acknowledgements

We would like to acknowledge the contribution, wisdom and insight of the people with learning disabilities whom we have worked with over the years. We thank them for their generosity in sharing their experiences of hope, pain and joy, and for teaching us the true meaning of resilience.

We would like to thank the many people who have helped us to produce this book. First to our colleagues on the BSc Integrated Practice in Learning Disability Nursing and Social Work programme, Noel Fagan, Valerie Houghton, Jenny Jones and Sarah Kennedy, all of whom contributed entries in respect of their specialist topics. To colleagues in health, social work, social care and third-sector services who have given their time freely to help us to sort out the reality from the rhetoric in terms of implementation of policy and legislation. To our students, past and present, who continue to inspire and challenge us every day. To colleagues at Palgrave, particularly Helen Caunce for encouraging us to produce the book in the first instance and to Peter Hooper and Louise Summerling whose patience and support have helped us to bring it to fruition.

Finally we would like to thank our families and friends for their continued support, endless reading of drafts and a plentiful supply of hot beverages, the latter of those things being (as fans of Sheldon Cooper will know) the cure-all for people in distress.

**Angela Olsen** would like to dedicate this book to her nephews Robert and Thomas Kemp and to Kelly Hunter who is a fantastic advocate for the rights of people with learning disabilities.

**Andrea Pepe** dedicates this book to Philipa, who has fought alongside people with learning disabilities and campaigned for their equality and rights for the last 30 years – her creativity, bravery and tenacity have always been an inspiration – and to Joey for his innate sense of fairness and inclusion, and occasionally emptying the dishwasher in times of stress.

**Dan Redfearn** dedicates this book to his late father, Michael, a brave man 'who fought against injustice, and struggled to be free' (Lunedei 1995). And to Louise, Jess and James, with much love.

# introduction

The term learning disability is complex and contested; indeed, some readers of this book may be surprised that we have used this term rather than the term intellectual disability. While the ***terminology*** entry discusses some of the issues surrounding the acceptability or otherwise of using specific labels to identify individuals or groups of people, our use here is in its broadest sense. We would ask readers to look beyond the words to consider the everyday experiences of people who for whatever reason are, in the main, still oppressed and marginalised in Britain in the 21st century.

We recognise that this book will not be accessible to a significant number of people with learning disabilities. This is by necessity, given the constraints of this type of book. However, it is written with the intention of highlighting pertinent issues, while promoting the rights, value, choice, independence and inclusion of people with learning disabilities. We have endeavoured to keep the voices of people with learning disabilities central to all our thinking and make no apologies for the strong ethical and values-based underpinning of this work. We remain committed to developing further accessible resources that are co-produced by people with learning disabilities in the future.

This book could easily have become a dictionary of syndromes and phenotypes. We have chosen to eschew the biomedical focus and concentrate instead on policy, practice and experiences relating to the lives of people with learning disabilities. However, some common syndromes have been included because large numbers of people with learning disabilities are affected by them. In these cases, we have endeavoured to focus on the social implications rather than the biomedical implications of the syndrome.

This book is designed to provide an overview of the current thinking and practice in key areas in the world of learning disabilities. It is intended to enhance interest, to promote understanding and to stimulate further reading rather than to provide a comprehensive one-stop resource.

We believe the content will be of interest and use to a wide range of people. This would include families, social workers, nurses, allied health professionals, social care workers, teachers, housing providers, police officers and others who live with and whose work brings them into contact with people who have learning disabilities.

Students and newly qualified practitioners across a range of disciplines will benefit from this text and can use it as an introduction to key concepts and issues with regard to people with learning disabilities. It might be of particular use to students in learning disability nursing or social work and to allied health professionals.

# how to use this book

The book is presented in alphabetical order, with each entry being a self-contained introduction to a topic related to learning disabilities. More observant readers will note that we have only offered an 'A to T' of learning disabilities and so cannot claim the book to be an exhaustive exploration of issues that affect people with learning disabilities. While it is not designed to be read in its entirety, readers are encouraged to identify topics of interest and use each entry as a reference point when issues arise in study or practice.

This book might most obviously be of use to learning disability practitioners; however, we believe it is also of importance to, and provides a helpful entry point for, other disciplines. An example might be an advocate who is supporting an individual with a housing issue who might find the ***accommodation*** entry helpful, or the entry on ***maternity and parenting*** might be of use to midwives or teachers who are working with parents who have a learning disability.

Each entry identifies *Implications for practice*, which are designed to summarise the entry, to help the reader to consider the impact in their own field of interest and to stimulate further research.

Suggestions for **FURTHER READING** are listed; these include web resources, journals and points of contact as well as traditional academic sources. Readers are encouraged to use these recommendations to enhance their knowledge and understanding, and to improve their practice and support of people with learning disabilities. Some of the resources are intended to be shared with people with learning disabilities and their families, for example the entry on ***siblings*** provides a link to Sibs, an organisation that supports families of people with disabilities. Every effort has been taken to ensure that where provided web resources are from stable sources and that all organisations recommended are in existence at the time of publication.

Further exploration of topics is also possible by readers utilising the references identified in the text of each entry, full details of which can be found in the reference list at the end of the book.

SEE ALSO sections at the top of each entry offer suggestions of related topics that readers can explore in order to broaden their knowledge of relevant issues. Some topics may not be understood in their entirety without reference to the SEE ALSO recommendation. For example the ***behaviour*** entry needs to be read in conjunction with the ***behavioural approaches*** entry.

# a

## accommodation

SEE ALSO **criminal justice; joint health and social care assessment framework; restrictive practice; serious case reviews; shared lives**

Historically most people with learning disabilities have lived at home with their parents. During the late 19th and for most of the 20th century, many were admitted to long-stay hospitals in isolated areas with little if any access to their families and communities. The hospital closure programme of the 1980s and 1990s resulted in people being returned to their local communities with many people 'resettled' in four to six-bedded houses in the same local authority as their families. Resettlements were usually managed by multi-agency resettlement teams including nurses, social workers and occupational therapists who tried to ensure that people lived with other residents or tenants that they were compatible with. In reality, the speed of the hospital closure programme led to people moving from large rural institutions to small urban institutions to spend the rest of their lives with people with whom they had little in common.

This model of housing has persisted, with many people continuing to live in houses along with other people with learning disabilities. Models of support and ownership of properties has changed significantly, with many people now occupying their own tenancies in housing association or private landlord lets, and receiving social care support from private or third-sector care agencies.

According to information gathered by local authorities and sent to the Health and Social Care Information Centre, approximately 74 per cent of the 140,015 adults with learning disability known to them are living in settled accommodation (Public Health England 2014). This includes independent and local authority provision as well as registered nursing care where support needs are higher and people live in usually small to medium-sized units where they are commonly 'placed' as a result of their higher support needs. The majority of people live with their families or other carers, and an increasing number have more individualised tenancies including ownership. Many are still supported by local authority or, increasingly, private companies' staff teams, but creative models of housing and support of people with learning disabilities are now developing across the country. A small percentage of individuals remain in acute and long-stay residential or hospital accommodation.

These figures do not account for the 26 per cent of people with learning disabilities living in what is considered to be risky accommodation, including sleeping rough or squatting, night shelters, emergency or direct access hostels, temporary homeless accommodation and refuges. While these figures relate to those 'known' to local authorities, the gap between this and estimated numbers of people with learning disabilities means that the number in 'risky' accommodation is likely to be much higher.

Other forms of accommodation include Intentional Communities; these generally offer a shared life experience. Such communities work under the ethos of people with learning disabilities and people without disabilities living together with equal status, sharing their lives without an acknowledged hierarchy of cared-for and carer. Originally situated in rural areas, although increasingly to be found in more urban areas, Intentional Communities such as Camphill Communities, L'Arche and the Home Farm Trust offer a degree of self-sufficiency in terms of growing food, providing education and employment. Many have a shared religious or spiritual belief. Supporters of such communities welcome the generally peaceful pace of life, the relative lack of threat often experienced in open communities – see entry on ***hate crime*** – and the equality between disabled and non-disabled inhabitants. Critics of this way of life suggest that people with learning disabilities are cut off from communities and that people without disabilities tend not to stay more than a year. Such a high turnover of support can be challenging for people who like routine.

Returning to those people with learning disabilities still supported in inpatient facilities, significant attention has been focussed on reducing the numbers in this form of accommodation following a number of major exposés such as those at Winterbourne

View (*Undercover Care* 2011) and Brompton Care Home (*MacIntyre Undercover* 1999) in programmes being broadcast on mainstream television. Both programmes revealed systematic ill treatment of people with learning disabilities by those who were paid to care for them.

Subsequent reports, most notably the *Winterbourne View – Time for Change* (Bubb 2014), challenged the practice of prolonged stays in assessment and treatment units for people with autism and mental health difficulties. The report introduced the requirement for an agreed discharge plan to be put in place from the point of admission, in an attempt to prevent people being admitted indefinitely. The report also introduced care and treatment review alongside the right for families to demand such reviews where they believe that assessment or treatment is not meeting the needs of their child.

The Bubb report built on the recommendations of preceding Mansell reports (1993 & 2007) which had called for the cessation of movement of people with challenging behaviour and mental health needs from their own local authorities to 'out of area' placements (OOA), and challenged housing providers to create better housing for people with complex needs.

The use of OOAs had been common practice for local authorities who have used them to respond to the needs of individual 'cases' rather than building up expertise in supporting people with complex needs. Such placements claimed to offer expertise in supporting challenging behaviour or providing adapted accommodation for people with complex health needs which may require access to lowered switches, adapted cookers and kitchen equipment and other assistive technologies for people who might rely on wheelchairs.

The report was followed in October 2015 with the announcement of a £45 million transformation plan, although on closer inspection this was not 'new' money, merely a re-focussing of monies already in the NHS and local authority budgets. The plan, *Building the right support: A national implementation plan to develop community services and close inpatient facilities*, proposed to close 50 per cent of assessment and treatment units by 2019. With a pledge to invest in local services for people who have learning disabilities and/or autism and behaviour that challenges services, the transformation plan proposed the clustering of clinical commissioning groups and reaffirmed the notion of pooling budgets with local authorities to invest in the development of community-based services. The plan copies the previous hospital closure programme by providing a dowry to local authorities to resettle people who have been in hospital the longest. The plan also details national guidelines so that people and their families will know what support and services they can expect.

*Implications for practice*

- Most people with learning disabilities are able to live in ordinary homes in ordinary communities and do not need specialist accommodation.
- The Care Act (2014) and *Building the right support* (Houlden 2015) both require the assessment of individual need and encourage the use of community resources to support people with learning disabilities.
- The first assumption must be that a person with a learning disability can be supported in an ordinary community, rather than being moved to a specialist facility.
- If a person is placed in a specialist assessment service, they should be given a date and clear plan for returning to their home community at the start of the assessment.
- Sir Stephen Bubb and Lynn Romeo (the Chief Social Worker for Adults) both assert the need for a Commissioner for learning disabilities. The role should be created outside of the NHS, allowing the post holder to hold health services to account for future improvements in healthcare.

**FURTHER READING**

- Housing and Support Alliance, www.housingandsupport.org.uk.

## adult social care services

SEE ALSO **care planning; healthcare services; joint health and social care self-assessment personalisation; professional practice**

Adult social care is a term used to describe the range of services provided for adults by local authorities. The term encompasses a range of strategic and developmental services such as overseeing the delivery of the autism strategy and Transforming Care programme and also includes social work and social care services.

The term social worker is a protected title in the UK, meaning that only people who have achieved the necessary qualifications and have registered with the Health and Care Professions Council can use the title social worker. Social work training is generic, equipping registrants to work with children and adults, people with disabilities and long-term health conditions, as well as those who are vulnerable or disadvantaged through other means, such as social deprivation, ethnicity, sexual or domestic violence, drug and substance misuse etc.

Social work roles are many and varied, including safeguarding adults and children, therapeutic interventions such as family work, drug and alcohol work and advocacy. Social workers might also contribute to the development of community social action groups to campaign for better opportunities for marginalised groups.

However, the most common task undertaken by social workers is that of assessment. Social workers have a legal duty to assess the needs of individuals who may be vulnerable due to age, disadvantage or disability and may need additional support to maintain wellbeing if the individual requests such an assessment.

Until recently, all adults with learning disabilities who asked for an assessment of need were assessed by social workers or other officers empowered by local authorities to do so. This began to change in 2009 with the introduction of a supported self-assessment tool called Resource Allocation System (RAS). The system, introduced by the Putting People First Concordat (Department of Health 2007), encourages people to assess their own level of need by answering a set of questions about their health, wellbeing and competence in completing daily living tasks. The RAS is intended to enable individuals to have more control over their own assessment. The fact that the system is long and complicated and has predetermined questions calls this into question, and many people have found it difficult to complete. In response to this, the Care Act 2014 placed a duty on local authorities to provide as much or as little support as the person needs to ensure that they get the best out of their assessment. In reality this means that many people with learning disabilities still rely heavily on the support of social workers to complete their RAS forms.

The RAS attaches points, which equate to funding, to aspects of health and support needs. The idea behind this approach is that people can predict the levels of financial support that they might receive. The RAS complements a move away from service provision and towards the provision of personal budgets (PBs), giving people more control over how they spend their time and money. An allocation of a PB can be used by a person to buy the type of support that best suits them and does not 'force' them to buy services that local authorities and others 'think' they might want.

Advocates of the system celebrate the fact that the PB can be used to fund any legitimate activity. For example, a person who is assessed as being isolated from their community and in need of mental and physical activity might have previously been allocated a place in a day centre for six hours each week. The equivalent PB might allow them to pay a personal assistant (PA) to go to a football match with them. Attending a football match might require physical activity to get to the match, perhaps helping a person to gain confidence in using public transport; it also enables a person to feel part of a community and can help them to make new friends who share a common interest, and lead to other activities. A day in a day centre is unlikely to meet these needs in such a positive way.

Critics highlight the potential monetisation of family relationships, citing instances of individuals paying family members as PAs. There are instances where families have prevented members with learning disabilities from moving out of the family home for fear of losing the PB or their own PA payments. It must be acknowledged, however, that social workers have long been aware of families who only appear to provide care and support for their relatives in order to maintain access to social security benefits.

The bulk of adult social care is provided by social care workers, not social workers. The term support worker is used to describe a range of occupational roles, including the PA role. This commonly involves a person directly employing PAs to meet their needs. It also includes those workers who might work for care agencies and make short visits to provide assistance with morning and bedtime routines. More structured support might be provided to people living in supported tenancies, where a team of workers provide round the clock support, assisting people with all aspects of daily living.

*Implications for practice*

- Adult social care is changing rapidly as more people have access to PBs.
- Public sector provision is set to continue to decline in number, as austerity cuts force local authorities to reduce service provision.

**FURTHER READING**

- Gray, A.M. & Birrell, D. (2013) *Transforming adult social care contemporary policy and practice* (Bristol: Policy Press).
- Care Quality Commission. (2015) *Guidance for adult social care providers*, www.cqc.org.uk/content/adult-social-care-providers.

## adulthood

SEE ALSO **empowerment; discrimination; hate crime; risk**

Being an adult is usually seen as a time of personal fulfilment where people are able to live independent lives and in the context of legal, economic and social constraints can make decisions to do as they wish. For people with learning disabilities, this is not always the case, and individual freedoms and choices are restricted further by their need for support, limitations placed on them by others, and by direct and indirect discrimination from individuals, groups, organisations and legal and societal structures. This means that people with learning disabilities are often not able to participate as full and active citizens in society or to achieve valued social roles (Wolfensberger 1998), leading to exclusion and isolation.

These restrictions must be understood and acknowledged when working with adults with learning disabilities, and the impact they may have on individuals must be considered. Some people might not recognise or seem affected by such restrictions, whereas others might see their non-disabled peers in valued social roles and aspire to do the same by getting a job or having a personal relationship, but they experience active discrimination in trying to achieve this (Williams 2009).

Regardless of the perception of the individual, any support of adults with learning disabilities must work to enhance their rights and promote independence and participation in society as valued citizens with the same opportunities as everyone else. Giving individuals choice and control over even small decisions enables them to develop a greater control over their lives and reduces the power and restrictions placed on them. Working in partnership with them empowers them with an equal relationship where you can work together to break down barriers and achieve goals and aspirations, which leads to better life experiences. This ethical approach is backed by clear government policy directives which identify a need for both individual and structural approaches to promote inclusion for people with learning disabilities, and it is important to engage with advocacy on all levels and in all settings.

*Implications for practice*

- Adults with learning disabilities should be involved in all decisions made about their care/treatment/support.
- All support should be concerned with the promotion of independence through choice and control.
- Person-centred approaches should be used in order to help adults with learning disabilities communicate and develop their dreams and aspirations, and to identify how these can be achieved.
- The rights of adults with learning disabilities should be promoted more widely through the development of awareness and challenge of discrimination, with the aim that individuals are regarded more positively.

**FURTHER READING**


- Kelly, A. (2001) *Working with adults with a learning disability* (Oxon: Speechmark Publishing).
- Thomas, D. & Woods, H. (2003) *Working with people with learning disabilities* (London: Jessica Kingsley Publishers).


## advocacy

SEE ALSO **empowerment; human rights and the disability movement; mental capacity**

Advocacy in all its forms seeks to ensure that people are able to speak out, to express their views and defend their rights. Effective advocacy enables someone to gain access to the things they need, to have a decent quality of life and to feel like a worthy and valued part of society. Without it, people disadvantaged by discrimination are often left feeling powerless and without a voice.

Fortunately, advocacy is supported by important and well-established legislation which ensures advocates have some power and leverage when it comes to representing peoples' rights. The concept of advocacy is underpinned by the Human Rights Act 1998, which introduced the notion of 'fairness' under Article 6: 'Right to a fair trial'. 'Fair' is taken to mean that a person has a right to present their case under conditions which do not place them at a substantial disadvantage when compared to the other party.

*Valuing People* (Department of Health 2001) supported the development of advocacy services for people with learning disabilities in recognition of the fact that their human rights were often compromised. It recommended that local authorities should work in partnership with third-sector services to provide specialist advocacy services for people with learning disabilities.

The Mental Capacity Act (2005) and the Mental Health Act (2007) both make provision for the use of advocates. The Mental Capacity Act introduced a new type of advocacy, the Independent Mental Capacity Advocate (IMCA). An IMCA provides advocacy in the event that there is no one who can be appropriately consulted when making a decision about a person deemed to not have mental capacity.

The Mental Health Act (2007) introduces the idea of Independent Mental Health Advocates who are available to people subject to the Mental Health Act, including people with learning disabilities who may also have mental health needs.

Advocacy seeks to ensure that people who are disenfranchised, disempowered and disadvantaged within society are supported to say what they want, secure their rights, represent their interests and obtain services they need (Empowerment Matters CIC & the National Development Team for Inclusion 2014).

Advocacy can be divided into two broad types. First, people who take action for themselves as individuals or groups; this is also known as **self-advocacy**, and organisations such as People First have groups that meet locally which are run by and for people with learning disabilities. Second, volunteers and paid professionals or **citizen advocates** are those who speak up on behalf of others who are unable to do so due to difficulties in communication, lack of capacity, discrimination or disempowerment.

Families also often act as advocates for a person with a learning disability, although this can be problematic if there is a conflict of interest. Professional advocacy also has its limitations where a worker may be constrained by statutory obligations, budgetary and organisational policies, procedural guidance and their code of practice.

Research has identified that the minority ethnic communities and people with profound and multiple health needs commonly have less access to advocates (Lawton 2009).

The need for advocacy services has increased with the personalisation agenda, personal care budgets and changes to NHS and GP commissioning; however, advocacy organisations report cuts in funding and insecure funding streams. It has also been argued that statutory advocacy may be funded at the expense of other types of advocacy (Action for Advocacy 2011).

*Implications for practice*

- When advocating on behalf of another person, the advocate must always take instruction from the client and act in their best interest.
- Many specialist advocacy services are closing due to cuts in public services. People with learning disabilities may still be able to seek support from organisations such as Welfare Rights services and Citizens Advice Bureaux.
- Practitioners need to ensure that people with learning disabilities have access to advocates as well as advocacy groups. It is vital that as far as possible people with learning disabilities are aware of their rights and empowered to have their own voice heard.

**FURTHER READING**


- Action for Advocacy. (2008) *Lost in translation: Towards an outcome focused approach to advocacy provision* (London: Action for Advocacy).
- Equality and Human Rights Commission. (2010) *Advocacy in social care for groups protected under equality legislation*, www.scie-socialcareonline.org.uk/advocacy-in-social-care-for-groups-protected-under-equality-legislation/r/a11G00000017zdnIAA.

- National Forum of People with Learning Difficulties. (2011) *Staying strong: Taking self-advocacy into the future*, www.nationalforum.co.uk/uploads/self_advocacy_guide_web_pdf.pdf.
- Bateman, N. (2000) *Advocacy skills for health and social care professionals* (London: Jessica Kingsley Publishers).


## ageing

SEE ALSO **dementia**

As with the general population, people with learning disabilities are living longer, and there is now evidence that suggests that people with 'mild' learning disabilities have a similar life expectancy to the general population (British Psychological Society 2015).

Bigby (2005) argues that the life experiences of people with learning disabilities significantly impact on their experience of growing older. An example of this is retirement; with the majority of people with learning disabilities not in employment (paid or voluntary), they will not usually follow this rite of passage that celebrates achievement and looks forward to an 'earned' more relaxed lifestyle. Other evidence, including the 'Growing Old With Learning Disabilities' project from the late 1990s (Wertheimer 2002), indicates that being forced to 'retire' from day centres and potentially moving from home with parents or supported living placements into older peoples services have a major impact on people's relationships, activity and emotional wellbeing.

The specific impact this may have on individuals is not clear; however, people with learning disabilities will continue to experience the same issues they may have faced throughout their lives such as increased health needs, poorer access to services, segregation and isolation, discrimination, lower expectations, fewer choices etc. (Bigby 2005). Many of these issues are often used in relation to the experience of older people more generally, and while there may be a risk of double discrimination on account of age and learning disability, the things that are important to people in older age may not be as different as some of the evidence suggests.

A small-scale study of people with learning disabilities who are 'growing older' identified that the most important things to them are being able to: speak up for themselves with someone taking the time to listen to them; have a home and live in safety; plan for the future; maintain close family links, relationships and friendships; have an active, healthy and fulfilling life; and face bereavement and the prospect of one's own death (Ward 2012). These ideas would not be too different to what most people would identify, and they can help to shape how people with learning disability are supported as they grow older.

*Implications for practice*

- Good support for people with learning disabilities as they age should not be substantially different to how they have been supported through their adult lives.
- An emphasis on person-centred approaches will mean that any specific emotional or psychological needs that arise should be accommodated along with an awareness of the potential for additional health needs.
- People should be supported to identify what is important for them in their older age and to have plans to ensure that this happens.

**FURTHER READING**

- British Institute of Learning Disabilities (ageing well information), www.bild.org.uk/information/ageingwell/.

## assessment

SEE ALSO **adult social care services; care planning**

### the process of assessment

The key to effective assessment is the recognition that it is a complex process that underpins both our understanding of the needs of individuals, groups or even communities that we support, and providing practitioners with core information that will shape the nature of any intervention.

In addition to needs identification, effective assessment also highlights the skills required by the practitioner to effectively support the individual; the resources needed to maximise the chances of successful outcomes; and the identification of experiences or opportunities that would enable the service user to engage and develop new skills or competencies that enhance their independence and quality of life.

In short, the key purpose of the assessment process is to set clear, unambiguous goals for the individual, group or community seeking support.

**criteria for effective assessment**

In order to ensure the efficacy of interventions, it is vital to ensure a number of key criteria:

- That the information collected is both valid and recent and accurately reflects the current rather than historical needs of the person. People who have learning disabilities are often assessed by others who carry with them negative assumptions that may lead to lowered expectations or even the presumption of failure to achieve.
- In relation to data collection, practitioners need to ensure that they are collecting focussed and relevant information and involve those best placed to collate that data. This may mean constructing data-gathering tools that are clear, unambiguous and accessible to parents or carers and the service user themselves.
- When entering the assessment process, it is essential that the practitioner does so with the aim of identifying actual rather than perceived needs and that objective evidence is sought rather than mere assumptions.
- In particular, the assessor needs to ensure that any assessment undertaken identifies the *strengths* of the individual as well as the *needs*. Too often there is a focus on what people can't do and a failure to recognise that they may have some interests, knowledge, experience and skills which can be used to help them to achieve their dreams.
- Having said that, effective assessment requires the establishment of clear baseline data so that there is confidence and clarity of the starting point.
- As part of the process of assessment, it is important to explore the range of options available to the practitioner, and the service user, in relation to achieving a successful outcome. In other words, could the need be met in a number of different ways?

- Finally, it is key to any future intervention that at this stage of the assessment, criteria for success are established so that it is known in advance when the intervention has been successful or whether there is a need to reassess if goals are not reached. These criteria need to be realistic and accurately reflect achievable outcomes for the person.

**barriers to effective assessment**

The process of assessment is often a complex procedure made more difficult by a number of common barriers. These include:

- Poor communication between and/or ineffective participation of all key members of the support team whether they be other professionals or family members and carers.
- Incomplete or inaccurate assessment data.
- Inconsistent collection of assessment data.
- Poor data-gathering processes.
- Inaccurate collection of data.

Each of these barriers can be overcome by adhering to the principles of effective assessment, but it is essential that, during the assessment period, practitioners are conscious of these potential pitfalls and actively monitor and support accurate collection and collation of assessment data.

As a practitioner supporting people with learning disabilities, the need to develop skills in assessment is clear. Practitioners must appreciate the purpose and process of assessment in relation to the provision of services and support. In addition, they need to understand the crucial role that effective communication can play in the process. Another key component of assessment is data management, including the need for analytical thinking and weighing of all *relevant* assessment data in order to reach a justifiable decision. The final stage of assessment is the identification and management of resources. Each of these elements contributes to the increased potential that the assessment and intervention result in positive outcomes for those receiving support.

Having considered the role of assessment in professional practice, there is also now a need to give consideration to the theories and models of assessment that guide practice, to consider how different approaches to the process can affect the outcome, and appreciate the central role that assessment can play in forming supportive relationships with users and carers.

It is important to bear in mind that assessment, as a process, should not be seen merely as a technical procedure that is too rigidly applied, irrespective of the person at the centre of that assessment. Assessment tools are just that – tools that can be used and applied skilfully and effectively by knowledgeable practitioners.

Neither is the assessment process value-free. Different approaches to the process should be used selectively, dependent on the needs as well as the preferences of the service user or carer. Effective assessment is the product of the mutual influence of the skilled practitioner AND the service user.

A number of the approaches to, and models of, assessment commonly referred to by practitioners in deciding how to conduct any given assessment task will be considered. In general terms, the three most common approaches outlined by Smale et al. (1993) are:

> The Questioning Model – As the name implies, this approach largely involves the practitioner posing a series of questions to the service user or carer. Generally seen as a very structured approach, the questions are often formulaic and predetermined by service providers. In this model, the practitioner is seen primarily as active and the user/carer as largely passive in shaping the outcome of the assessment. The influence of the practitioner is significant, being perceived as the 'expert' and in the position to both interpret and define the information and define the 'problem' as well as the outcome. Despite the potential imbalance in power and influence innate in this model, it may well have a role in practice. For instance, it is a useful approach to adopt in situations such as risk assessment or in the event of an emergency referral. However, its limits need to be recognised, as it clearly restricts the participation of service users and carers.
>
> The Procedural Model – In this approach, the practitioner uses organisational guidelines or checklists to complete the assessment. Such guidance or formats are often designed to fit the agency criteria for access to support or services. Once again, the 'expert' in this approach is a professional, in this case the

author or designer of the guidance or assessment format, and the practitioner is simply collecting information predetermined by others. Such assessment tools cover a very broad range of needs experienced by people with learning disabilities, ranging from sleep or continence assessments through to highly complex tools designed to identify factors that impact on mental health or behaviours that challenge. As this model is frequently used for formal or statutory assessments, it is important to recognise that the outcome is possibly influenced by a constraint on resources, and this may introduce the concept of meeting an eligibility criteria set in advance. However, it is equally important to recognise that such structured assessments do make the collection of factual and objective information possible, though it risks missing out on the subjective thoughts or feelings of the user or carer.

The Exchange Model – In this approach, there is a much more equitable balance of power between the practitioner and the user/carer. In its purest form it may even be accepted that the user, or their carer, is in fact the 'expert'. Here the practitioner empowers and enables the user to identify strengths and interests as well as needs, and facilitates the user to take more control of the assessment process and problem resolution. This approach does not ignore the inevitable power imbalance that still exists between providers and users but recognises it and aims to manage it. Clearly there are challenges, and perhaps limitations, associated with this approach in that empowering those with the most complex needs in the assessment process poses particular problems for practitioners. Nonetheless, these are challenges that should be accepted enthusiastically, and all possible means of achieving more equitable partnership working should be sought.

**empowerment in the assessment process**

In order to identify strategies to further empower people with learning disabilities in the process of assessment, there is a need to start by reflecting on the origin and source of practitioner power in the therapeutic relationship (Smale et al. 1993). For anyone encountering any professional practitioner, there is often the notion of the 'expert' having a pool of knowledge, skills and expertise not held by the layperson. The professional also has experience and knowledge of processes and procedures, of 'how the system works', which is often a mystery to service users and their carers. Professionals tend to use lots of jargon that is understood by them alone but is almost a foreign language to those outside the profession. Finally, for an individual service user or carer to be faced by a whole team of professionals can be very intimidating.

There are a number of practical strategies that can be successfully adopted that would increase the degree of influence of users and carers in the assessment process and thus challenge the power balance:

- Consider practical changes such as identifying more appropriate venues, times and formats of meetings to discuss assessments that best suit the needs of the user.
- Allow sufficient preparation time for service users prior to any formal discussion or meeting.
- Retain the focus of the assessment process on the person rather than the situation that gave rise to the referral.
- Give proper recognition to strengths before addressing deficits or needs.
- Give equal weighting to alternative sources of assessment data such as personal accounts and preferences alongside formal assessment material.
- Ensure inclusive decision-making processes.
- Provide accessible assessment material, support plans and recording methods.
- Have open systems for sharing and monitoring developments during the assessment period.
- Show proper and mutual respect to alternative and perhaps competing perspectives in establishing assessment goals.

*Implications for practice*

- The views of the service user must always be central to any decision that is made with them or on their behalf.
- Practitioners must be able to draw on a range of assessment tools and techniques in order to undertake effective assessment.
- Social care services now encourage adults with learning disabilities to take control of their own assessments using the Resource Allocation System.

**FURTHER READING**

- Manthorpe, J., Alaszewski, A., Gates, B., Ayer, S. & Motherby, E. (2003) Learning disability nursing (*Journal of Intellectual Disabilities* 7(2): pp. 119–135).
- Milner, J., Myers, S. & O'Byrne, P. (2015) *Assessment in social work,* (London: Palgrave).
- Smale, G., Tuson, G. & Statham, D. (2000) *Social work and social problems* (London: Macmillan).
- Turnbull, J. (Ed.) (2004) *Learning disability nursing* (Oxford: Blackwell Science).

## assistive technology

SEE ALSO **accommodation; communication; physical disabilities; profound and multiple learning disabilities; sensory disabilities**

Assistive technology is an umbrella term that includes a range of devices used to support people with disabilities. The term can include medical devices such as hearing aids, wheelchairs, prosthetics and orthotics. Orthotics are aids such as limb and trunk braces that help to train or maintain posture and gait. Functional orthotics are those prescribed by an orthopaedic surgeon or physiotherapist and are customised to meet individual need. Assistive technology can also include accessible software to enhance the use of computing equipment, including laptops and smartphones to aid communication. The emphasis behind any assistive technology is that it promotes greater independence as well as health and social wellbeing.

### communication

Communication aids have a long history. Braille, a system of raised dots developed to assist blind people to read, is perhaps the method most familiar to the public. Other systems have been developed to assist different groups of people. The picture exchange communication system, commonly referred to as PECS, is a library of pictures that a person with autism or other communication difficulties carries with them, or has access to at home or school. Pictures are given to the person that they wish to communicate with, for example a child with limited speech will give their parent or teacher a picture of an apple to indicate a preference in choice of fruit at mealtimes. The picture will be returned to the child together with the apple.

Other examples of assistive communication tools include the BIGmack communicator, which allows people with profound and multiple learning disabilities to play specially recorded sounds and messages up to two minutes in length at the push of a button. These preloaded messages provide a quick and easy method of expressing simple, frequently used questions and responses.

The right to communication or 'a voice' is a fundamental human right often denied to people with learning disabilities as it often involves an investment of time and money. The purchase of assistive communication technology is not a priority for local authority or health service funders, so people are often left without a method of communicating effectively, leading to a misunderstanding of their needs by parents and support workers. This can lead to frustration on the part of both and can result in behaviour that is considered challenging.

The Royal College of Speech and Language Therapists launched the 'Giving Voice' Campaign in 2012 to highlight the need for such support to be made available by right. Initially designed to support the communication needs of people with dementia, the campaign has highlighted the need to improve communication support for people with learning disabilities as well.

**postural support**

The lives of many profoundly disabled people have been transformed by developments in orthotics and wheelchair technology. A powerful example of such developments can be seen in the cases of people with very limited upper body strength. Previously this condition would have meant that people had to endure lives spent lying prone on domestic versions of hospital trolleys. The development in orthotics to support the upper body means that people can now be supported in a sitting position in specially designed wheelchairs. The effect of raising a person from a recumbent to a sitting position is not only physiologically beneficial, improving breathing, digestion, blood flow etc., but it is also psychologically important as it brings the individual closer to eye level with other people.

John O'Brien, the author of Ordinary Life Principles (see entry on ***service philosophies***), showed the transformation in public attitudes when a young man that he knew moved from the prone position to being seated in a wheelchair. He showed pictures of the young man in both positions to a class of university students. The reactions to the photograph of the individual in the recumbent position included assuming: that the man was much younger than he was; that he had no verbal communication; and that he was completely helpless. Many students likened him to a baby. Reactions to the same man seated in a wheelchair were much more optimistic: students were much closer to reality in guessing his age; there was no suggestion that he was as dependent as a baby; and, indeed, he was assumed to have capacity to make decisions.

**housing**

Housing developers have been incentivised to design and build housing that supports the needs of people who use wheelchairs or have sensory disabilities. This is achieved by making them more accessible with larger doorways, ramps instead of steps, lower kitchen work surfaces; accessible bathrooms etc. Most people with learning disabilities, however, do not live in new-build houses and the cost of adapting their existing homes to enable them to move around safely can be enormous.

Disabled facilities grants are available for the adaptation of bathrooms, installation of stair lifts etc., but these are not available for smaller but equally important changes to support aspects of daily living.

Other technologies use a system of sensors and alarms, often referred to as 'Telecare', to help promote and maintain independence by allowing an individual to live in their own home but with safeguards to maintain safety in the event of an identified risk. When such an event happens, the sensors connect to a help centre or directly to carers who can take appropriate action to provide any required support. Examples include: a pendant alarm that the individual can wear round their neck and set off should they fall; a sensor to alert others when a door is opened, particularly late at night when the person is at risk of 'wandering'; or a mat that monitors for seizure activity for someone with epilepsy when they are sleeping.

Some significant developments have been achieved in recent years thanks to the advent of smartphones and associated technologies. Developers have created applications that enable people to switch their heating and lighting and other appliances on and off safely and easily. They can also monitor security in and around the home in terms of intrusion and also smoke, fire or gas emissions. Smartphones can be digitally operated or voice activated, and the cost of adapting existing homes to become smartphone-assisted homes is very attractive when compared with other options such as moving home or physically moving plugs or lights, relocating heating controls etc.

*Implications for practice*

- Assistive technologies can make a huge difference in the lives of people with disabilities; however, the provision of such technologies is not prioritised by local authorities.
- Developments in digital technology are advancing quickly; practitioners must keep abreast of such developments and support people in asserting their rights to be adequately supported in order to ensure their wellbeing.

**FURTHER READING**

- Aidis Trust, www.aidis.org.
- ATiA, www.atia.org.

## autism

SEE ALSO **communication; fragile x; mental health; sensory disabilities**

Autism is commonly linked to learning disabilities, although it is increasingly understood that a significant proportion of people on the autism spectrum do not have accompanying learning disabilities (Emerson & Baines 2010a).

Autism is often seen as a complex and unusual condition, at least in part due to the wide range of terms used to diagnose and refer to it. Autism (high or low functioning), Asperger syndrome, Childhood Autism, and Pervasive Developmental Disorder Not Otherwise Specified are just some of the labels which have been used, often interchangeably, causing confusion and misunderstanding.

Key autism representative groups and the UK government now commonly use 'autism' as an umbrella term for all such conditions, with 'autism spectrum disorders' or 'conditions' (ASC) also recognised as overarching descriptors of a range of previously separate terms that share significant features.

This broader understanding of autism is reflected in recent changes to the diagnostic criteria in *DSM-V* (American Psychiatric Association 2013). This removes previous individual diagnostic categories such as Asperger syndrome and replaces them with 'Autism Spectrum Disorders'. These changes also indicate that any diagnosis should focus on identifying the needs that an individual has resulting from the condition, and the extent to which these impact on their life and functioning.

While there are a number of common features experienced by people with autism, as the term spectrum suggests, individual experience may be very different with characteristics presented in different ways. Donna Williams (1996) perhaps explains this best from the perspective of an individual with autism, stating that it is:

> A range of ways of experiencing yourself and the world, of processing information about yourself and the world, of relating to yourself and the world which is different to that experienced by other people.

In both the new and more traditional diagnostic criteria (still defined in the *ICD-10* (World Health Organization 1992)), these differences are described as functional difficulties with: social communication; social interaction; and flexibility of thought often characterised by restricted and repetitive patterns of behaviour. These were described by Wing & Gould (1979) as the 'Triad of Impairment', with subsequent understandings also recognising that sensory-perceptual anomalies are a significant feature for many people with ASC (Boucher 2009).

A person with an ASC may have difficulties with both expressive and receptive communication, which can make understanding and interpretation problematic. There may be a distinctive rhythm or monotone to the voice, with a propensity for over-formulaic construct, repetitive questioning or echolalia. Receptive features may include a difficulty in processing both verbal and nonverbal information, with a tendency for literal interpretation and a focus on content over meaning.

As with the spectrum as a whole, the extent to which difficulties may be evident in an individual can vary from someone who is very articulate, to someone who is nonverbal, or who relies on vocalisations/alternative communication systems such as the use of pictures or symbols. However well a person can communicate, it tends to be functional rather than social, and the individual may have difficulty expressing wants, needs and particularly emotion.

Implicit in the act of communication is a level of social interaction which the majority of people with autism find very stressful. This can make an individual appear indifferent or passive, and they may choose to isolate themselves, usually due to the difficulties and misunderstandings experienced. When interaction does take place, there may be unusual eye contact, inappropriate responses, unusual behaviours (overbearing, passive, mannerisms) or the misunderstanding of social rules such as topic maintenance, turn-taking or the over-emphasis on their own interests to the exclusion of others.

When describing difficulties with flexibility of thought, we might think in terms of any cognitive function that allows us to process, explain, predict or interpret. This relates closely to psychological understandings of 'Theory of Mind' and 'Central Coherence' and may impact on an individual's ability to organise, generalise (meaning and skills), cope with change, perceive another person's point of view or have insight into their own difficulties. This can result in a reliance on routine or a focus on particular topics or interests that create a sense of familiarity and security.

Sensory-perceptual anomalies have increasingly been recognised as helpful in understanding the experience of an individual with autism. Anomalies can affect any or all of the senses (including proprioceptive and vestibular) and can present as either a deficit (hyposensitivity) or an extreme (hypersensitivity). The resulting impact can lead to an appearance of disinterest or the seeking out of sensory experience in the case of hyposensitivity, or distress, overload and withdrawal in the case of hypersensitivity. It is therefore important to try and understand the impact of sensory factors on an individual with autism's experience of communication, interaction and flexible thinking.

Given the potential difficulties with understanding and processing communication and interaction, it is perhaps unsurprising that many people with autism describe significant anxiety (especially in social situations), with an increased vulnerability to other mental health conditions also evident. Raised anxiety levels can lead to an increase in some of the 'behaviours' associated with the condition such as an increased reliance on routine, or preoccupation with special interests as a way of controlling tension and alleviating its impact.

Until recently, prevalence of ASCs was largely based on studies of childhood populations and the identification of 'autistic characteristics' within defined groups (Baird et al. 2006). Alongside the publication of the Autism Act (2009) and the National Strategy for Adults with Autism (Department of Health 2010), the UK government commissioned a prevalence study for adults (Brugha et al. 2012) which supported the figures previously identified. Both these studies suggest a prevalence rate of 1:100 or 1 per cent of the population. It is important to note that given the individual nature of experiences of autism, there will be a wide range of presenting needs requiring varying levels of support, or none.

Despite significant research, the exact cause of autism is still not known. It is commonly understood that genetic factors are the largest contributing factor (NHS Choices 2014), but no specific genes have been identified and it is likely the result of a complex set of genetic mutations, perhaps combined with external environmental factors or triggers. What is known is that autism is not the result of the MMR vaccination, or poor parenting. In a minority of cases, autism is a secondary feature of another syndrome or medical condition such as Fragile X. There is no simple 'test' to determine likelihood or presence of autism, and there is no 'cure'.

There has been much debate as to whether Asperger syndrome should be considered a condition in its own right or as part of the autism spectrum, but it is now commonly understood to be a form of autism and is included as part of all the major literature and legislation concerning autism, including the Autism Act (2009).

Asperger syndrome refers to a clinical grouping first described by Hans Asperger in 1944 and later named and further explored by Lorna Wing (1981), one of the leading writers and researchers of developmental disorders, particularly autism.

A person with Asperger syndrome will share many of the same characteristics as someone with autism, particularly in relation to the key functional difficulties highlighted above. This means that engaging and understanding communication and interaction can be challenging, and there may be evidence of routines, repetitive activities, resistance to change and a narrow field of interests, as well as sensory-perceptual anomalies.

Where Asperger syndrome has often been seen to differ is in a perception of characteristics being 'less obvious' to the observer – although significant difficulties may still be experienced by the individual.

Many of these differences are more marked through the developmental stages of childhood where a child with autism may have delayed development of speech; the child with Asperger syndrome has no delay at all. Despite these subtler differences, as part of the autism spectrum, the core elements remain the same, with people with Asperger syndrome typically having fewer problems with speaking and language and fewer accompanying learning disabilities.

As previously highlighted, the category of Asperger syndrome has now been removed from one of the leading diagnostic reference texts (American Psychiatric Association 2013), with the focus now on understanding how the condition impacts upon the individual and the resulting difficulties. While this change has been largely welcomed, the removal of individual diagnoses has caused negative reaction from some people, particularly with Asperger syndrome, who have a built sense of their own identity and membership of a community based on being an 'Aspie'.

In 2009, the Autism Act became the first disability-specific piece of legislation in UK history. This placed a duty on the government to produce a national strategy for adults with autism, which followed in 2010 when *Fulfilling and rewarding lives: The strategy for adults with autism in England* (Department of Health 2010) and accompanying statutory guidance to support its implementation was published.

The overall aim of the strategy was for people with autism to 'live within a society that accepts and understands them', with access to diagnosis and support from mainstream services. It set out guidance for developments in five key areas:

- Increased awareness and understanding across all public services.

- Development of a clear, consistent pathway for diagnosis and assessment.
- Improved access to services and support for independent living.
- Help for adults with autism to find and maintain employment.
- Strategic planning and development of local services.

The strategy was reviewed and updated in 2014 when *Think autism* was published (Department of Health 2014a). This update reinforced the requirements of the original strategy and statutory guidance while identifying 15 priority challenges for action to ensure people can be an equal part of their communities, get the right support at the right time and develop skills and independence to work to the best of their abilities. *Think autism* also proposes three specific action areas: to build autism awareness in communities through recognition of good practice and autism 'champions'; the introduction of an autism innovation fund to support projects that promote independence in the community; and to have more effective data collection, advice and information for people with autism. This strategy is due to be reviewed and updated in 2019.

*Implications for practice*

- Autism will affect each individual in a different way, and so it is important to work with them and those who know them well to understand the needs that they have resulting from the condition, and the extent to which this impacts on their lives.
- It is often as much about those around the individual understanding and supporting them effectively as it is about 'changing' them to fit in with societal expectations.
- Support should be developed to promote independence and community participation as equal citizens.
- Developing awareness of autism in the community is also vital.

## FURTHER READING

- *Autism: The International Journal of Research and Practice*. Sage Publications.
- Boucher, J. (2009) *The autistic spectrum: Characteristics, causes and practical issues* (London: Sage Publications).

- Department of Health. (2010) *Fulfilling and rewarding lives: The national strategy for adults with autism* (London: DH).
- Department of Health. (2014) *Think autism: An update to the government adult autism strategy* (London: DH).
- National Autistic Society, www.autism.org.uk.

# b

## behaviour

SEE ALSO **behavioural approaches; discrimination; restrictive practices**

Some people with learning disabilities are said to display 'challenging behaviour', but in reality this term relates to only 10–15 per cent of people with learning disabilities (Emerson 2001). Recent approaches have attempted to reframe the understanding of such behaviour in order to better understand an individual's presentation, to provide more effective support. However people within this group are still at significant risk of being detained in 'assessment and treatment' hospitals, with 2600 learning disability inpatients across the UK in 2014/15 (Bubb 2014).

When talking about challenging behaviour, people will commonly associate this with destructive, aggressive and violent behaviours such has hitting, kicking, biting etc. directed towards other people, property or the individual themselves (self injury). A wider understanding also incorporates socially inappropriate (including sexualised and obsessive) behaviours, resistance to tasks or demands, non-engagement and stereotyped behaviour such as rocking or echolalia (repeating the last words heard).

Emerson's 1995 definition of what should be classed as challenging behaviour is still commonly accepted as the preferred understanding:

> Behaviour of such intensity, frequency or duration that the physical safety of the person or others is likely to be placed in serious jeopardy, or behaviour which is likely to seriously limit use of, or result in the person being denied access to, ordinary community facilities. (Emerson 1995, p. 4)

While this has limitations in terms of subjectivity, the key aspect is the latter part of the definition, which places the emphasis on the negative outcomes for the individual rather than the direct consequences of the behaviour itself. This fits in with the broader approach to understanding behaviour that is described here.

Historically it has been assumed that 'challenging behaviour' results directly from an individual's learning disability, which has meant that other potential causes have not been acknowledged or explored, a process referred to as 'diagnostic overshadowing'. This has led to a misunderstanding of need and inappropriate support; however, more recent approaches are based on the principles that all behaviours have a function, and that they are socially defined.

Any behaviour is an attempt to engage with, control or manipulate the environment and situations that we face. For example the function of putting the kettle on to make a cup of tea is to meet our physical need for hydration, our emotional preference for tea and perhaps our social need for interaction with others.

When considering the function of behaviours that might be deemed challenging, there are a number of factors that might be seen as causing the behaviour, either in isolation or combination:

- Biological: some behaviours are features of specific syndromes associated with learning disabilities (Lesch Nyan – self injury; Prader-Willi – persistent feeling of hunger leading to constant eating).
- Physical: a person's behaviour may indicate that they are unwell or in pain, for example, if a person begins to hit themselves around the face or head, it is possible that they have toothache. It may also be a result of sensory imbalance.
- Social: an individual may engage in behaviours as they are bored, lacking in social interaction or they are unaware of expected behaviour in given situations.
- Environmental: behaviour could be a response to noises, lighting, temperature, crowds or other people.
- Psychological: the individual may be distressed, angry, frustrated, devalued or disempowered.

In addition to the factors detailed above, the behaviour may also be the individual's way of attempting to communicate their experience or feelings about what is happening to them or in their environment. Much of the emphasis in supporting someone with their behaviour should therefore be to understand what they are telling us.

In the same way that behaviour has a function, so each is judged in relation to the context in which it takes place. For example hitting someone with no provocation in the street might be deemed inappropriate and therefore 'challenging', whereas in the context of a boxing match it is accepted and celebrated as sporting prowess. Judgements are also subjective, based on a personal experience (i.e. what one person may view as challenging another may not) and in different social/cultural contexts.

This contextual understanding prompts us to consider why the individual is engaging with that behaviour at that specific time. Similar to the functions of behaviour, there may be a range of possible reasons: they may be trying to communicate; to initiate interaction; to avoid a specific situation or demand; or to fulfil some stimulatory deficit. Rather than just assuming the person's behaviour is directed towards a specific target, it is vital to consider the context of the behaviour in order to determine what action we should take.

Behaviours do not occur in isolation, and each is subject to a process of reinforcement depending on the response that has been elicited; however, once we begin to understand behaviour in this way, we change from viewing the problem or the challenge as being rooted in the individual to seeing it as a product of their environment, their situation, their needs not being adequately met and their communication of this. This should change our approach to intervention to ensure that all the individual's needs are met, thus reducing the need for the behaviour to occur (this will be considered further in the entry on ***behavioural approaches***).

*Implications for practice*

- When supporting people with learning disabilities who present with behaviours that may be deemed to challenge, it is vital to consider their context, purpose and function rather than just focussing on the effects or negative outcomes.
- Develop an understanding of the individual and their needs to inform effective support, which reduces the need for behaviours.
- Do not to try to change behaviours by punitive methods.

**FURTHER READING**

- Challenging Behaviour Foundation, www.challengingbehaviour.org.uk.
- Emerson, E. & Einfeld, S.L. (2011) *Challenging behaviour*, 3rd edition (Cambridge: Cambridge University Press).
- *Journal of Applied Behaviour Analysis*. Wiley Publications.

## behavioural approaches

SEE ALSO **behaviour; empowerment; personalisation; person-centred approaches; restrictive practice**

There has been a significant shift in the way that people with behaviours that challenge are supported over the last 20 years. Historical approaches focussed on the 'problem behaviour' and rooted this within the individual. Intervention was targeted towards changing or modifying behaviour, and managing or controlling it if this did not work. More recent approaches look at the wider context of the person in their environment and situation, with support based on understanding their behaviour to ensure that all needs are met. This is reflective of more fundamental changes in values towards people with learning disabilities that have been informed by the social model of disability, principles of normalisation and person-centred thinking.

Theories of psychological development and behavioural science have been at the forefront of working with people whose behaviour is deemed to be challenging. These theories have often utilised techniques that are based on behaviourist theories of learning, particularly 'operant' conditioning (Slevin 2007), which seek to understand and modify behaviour using principles of reinforcement. Techniques that fall within these methods have often been found to be unethical, as they have been based on aversive or punitive reinforcement.

Current thinking and practice emphasises that individuals should be supported within the framework of Positive Behavioural Support (PBS). Rather than being a model of behaviour management with a clear set of tools and methods, PBS is a much broader conceptual framework that is rooted in person-centred approaches to effectively support and increase personal skills, capabilities and competence while enhancing community presence and participation (Gore et al. 2013). This allies with a constructional approach where a reduction of challenging behaviour is a 'side effect' of increased skills and capacities. Where intervention is required, the emphasis is on proactive and preventative approaches to prevent and manage behaviours that challenge in an ethical, safe and effective way, rather than simply trying to control or manage problem behaviours.

PBS is a system-based approach that attempts to understand the behaviour in its wider environmental and social context. This will usually include elements of functional analysis, an approach fundamental to applied behavioural analysis, which seeks to assess why the person displays a particular behaviour. PBS emphasises a strong values base which avoids punitive interventions and instead focusses on understanding and manipulating setting conditions (personal and environmental factors such as stress or a lack of control, which make a behaviour more or less likely) and triggers (what provokes the behaviour at a given time) in order to reduce occurrence. At the same time, an emphasis is on developing alternative adaptive responses, including functionally equivalent behaviours (e.g. using a communication aid to indicate anxiety/wanting to leave rather than hitting someone, knowing the outcome would be removal). At the heart of PBS is the creation of suitable environments and services based on person-centred support, promoting the rights and developing skills of individuals.

In order to promote intervention that is rooted within PBS, a number of models have been utilised to help support an understanding of an individual's behavioural presentation and direct appropriate support. One of these is based on Kaplan & Wheeler's (1983) 'assault cycle', now more commonly known as the 'cycle of emotional arousal'. While this looks specifically at a person's physical and emotional responses to identified triggers, it is based on the assumption that all behavioural incidents are a deviation from a person's normal, or **baseline** emotional state (phases of this cycle are identified in bold). Underpinned by a holistic assessment, good general support should therefore be focussed on using preventative and proactive measures that ensure a person's needs are met and that they have the necessary skills and capacities that mean that behaviours are not required (e.g. all needs are met, new functional skills are taught, relationships are improved, communication is enhanced, access to activities and choices is provided etc.)

Deviation from the baseline is usually in response to a **trigger** which can be an internal (within the person) or external (in the environment or from other people) feeling, event, situation etc. At this point, proactive and responsive interventions can be combined to prevent **escalation** where a person's agitation levels increase and a more extreme behavioural response is more likely. De-escalation techniques can include distraction, redirection to a different activity or space, prompting positive appraisal of situations, removal from the trigger (or the trigger from the person) or relaxation techniques such as deep breathing or mindfulness. Good support in these phases will include recognition of potential and actual triggers, and taking appropriate steps to reduce the likelihood of them occurring and minimising their impact through knowing the individual and what de-escalation techniques they are likely to respond to.

If de-escalation fails, then the individual may reach **crisis**, at which point the behaviour is at its most extreme and intervention to prompt the person to calm is not likely to be effective. In this phase it is important to respond in an ethical way while maintaining the safety of all involved, including the individual displaying the behaviour, and to protect their dignity as much as possible. Intervention may include: a calm, rational response, having a safe and quiet place available, removing the person from the situation etc., but may also include restrictive practices which should only be a last resort and in line with the principles identified in the entry on ***restrictive practice***. All interventions should be planned and reviewed with lessons learned and implemented into future support.

The cycle of emotional arousal is helpful in prompting appropriate support following incidents where a person has had a crisis situation. It identifies a period of at least 90 minutes following an incident where a person remains physically and emotionally aroused and could easily respond to additional triggers with a further escalation of behaviour and possible crisis. This **recovery** phase is where mistakes can easily be made in support provided to the individual by asking them to rationalise their behaviour, or placing too many demands on them. Instead, a calm, low stimulus approach should be taken, ensuring the person's safety and offering support and reassurance as directed by them.

Following the recovery phase, a person is likely to experience **post-crisis depression** where the physical and emotional stresses of the incident have subsided and they regress below their normal baseline. In this phase, mental and physical exhaustion is common and the person may display guilt, shame or remorse, and so support should be focussed on relieving this through reassurance and helping the person understand and process the incident.

The cycle of emotional arousal, and other similar models, can be used as a framework for a positive behavioural care plan with identification of what a person's presentation is at each stage of the cycle, what is likely to impact on their emotional arousal, and the steps that should be taken at each stage in response. These principles also underpin governmental guidance for supporting the reduction of restrictive practices for individuals in learning disability and mental health settings detailed in *Positive and Proactive Care* (Department of Health 2014b) and *A Positive and Proactive Workforce* (Skills for Care 2014).

There has been considerable debate in the use of medication as a long-term therapeutic intervention to reduce or control behaviours that challenge, despite there being little evidence to support its effectiveness for this purpose (this is very different to use of medication at the point of crisis where other interventions have not been effective – see entry on ***restrictive practice***).

Evidence suggests that the number of people with learning disabilities prescribed psychotropic medication (used to treat certain mental health conditions) is far in excess of the number of people who have an actual mental illness (Sheehan et al. 2015) which seems to confirm concerns that they are often used inappropriately to supress or control symptoms (behaviour) rather than address the potential causes.

Rarely is medication utilised within a dimensional approach where the behaviour is known, or understood, to be resulting from specific deficits/excesses of brain function, for example serotonin or dopamine production. In these cases, medication can be targeted to stabilise hormone levels and therefore reduce the occurrence of behaviours. Similarly, if the underlying cause of the behaviour is depression, psychoses or another physical or mental condition for which medication is a recognised therapeutic intervention, then this should be used and consequentially should reduce the behaviours.

There may be a place for the use of medication in certain circumstances, but it should not be used as the first option and, in accordance with National Institute for Health and Clinical Excellence (NICE) guidelines, only when other interventions or treatments for coexisting conditions have not produced any change, or where the risk to the person or others is 'very severe' (NICE 2015). Even in these circumstances, medication should be considered a short-term option with other interventions established to taper the medication away.

Whenever medication is used, in whatever context, it should be carefully monitored for effects and side effects and reviewed to ensure it is not prescribed for longer than is clinically necessary.

For over 20 years, recommendations for supporting people with behaviours that challenge have centred on individually designed services based on a thorough assessment and understanding of the person so staff working with them have a detailed knowledge of how best to support them (Mansell 1993). While there are some examples of where this has been achieved through personalisation, service provision is more common in group settings and for individuals with more complex needs in institutional units, where an estimated 3500 people were still supported in early 2016 (Bubb 2016). This report again highlights that services should be community-based, with appropriate housing, suitably skilled and trained staff, and effective early intervention and prevention services to support people effectively in their communities.

*Implications for practice*

- Punitive and aversive behaviour modification techniques should not be used in the support of people with learning disabilities.
- Support should not just focus on an individual's behaviour, but on developing personal skills, capabilities and competence while enhancing community presence and participation.
- Intervention should be informed by a detailed assessment including a focus on the function or purpose of specific behaviours with responses to prevent, de-escalate or manage them identified in a plan of care.
- Medication should only be used where there is a clear purpose and process for monitoring and review.

- People working and supporting individuals with behaviours that challenge should have access to high-quality training in PBS and how to provide ethical support and intervention.

## FURTHER READING


- British Institute of Learning Disabilities, www.bild.org.uk.
- Challenging Behaviour Foundation, www.challengingbehaviour.org.uk.
- *The International Journal of Positive Behaviour Support*, BILD Journals.
- Hardy, S. & Joyce, T. (2011) *Challenging behaviour: A handbook: Practical resource addressing ways of providing positive behavioural support to people with learning disabilities whose behaviour is described as challenging* (Brighton: Pavilion Publishing).

# C

## care planning

SEE ALSO **assessment; behaviour; behavioural approaches; interprofessional practice; person-centred approaches**

Any person supported by services, including people who have a learning disability, should have a care plan that guides the support and intervention that they receive. These take many different forms, from those required by law in order to inform the statutory provision of services (such as those under the Care Act 2014), to plans that support specific aspects of care, such as a person's day-to-day support, behaviour that may challenge, or an identified health need within a nursing care plan.

Care plans are part of the 'process' of care (Sutton 2006). They are informed by an assessment that identifies what support is needed and then details how it will be provided. A good assessment and care plan should not just account for the presenting 'need' of the individual, but should look at this within the individual's wider context, be developed in consultation with them and, where appropriate, with their support network, including family, friends, paid members of support staff and the wider multidisciplinary team.

The care plan can be described as an 'instruction manual' for the support or intervention an individual requires. It should detail:

- *What* will be done.
- *How* it will be done.
- *Who* it will be done by (e.g. the service user, social worker, support staff, nurse etc.).
- *When* it is going to be done.
- Plans for review against the expected outcomes.

Care plans should support and guide the individual, as much as those who are giving support, and should include what is important to them and any goals that they want to work towards. Goals need to be realistic, with identified targets towards their achievement. Care plans may also be used to inform the 'purchase' of services when an individual has an assessment under the Care Act 2014 and a care manager is procuring services to meet identified needs.

Returning to the 'process' of care, plans should not be static and unchanging but should be subject to ongoing review both formally (at specified intervals, e.g. 3, 6, 12 months) and informally (if something changes in the period between reviews, this should be addressed in consultation with the individual and their support network, and not left until the plan is due for review). This promotes the ongoing 'process' of support, with assessment/evaluation happening at every stage to inform the planning and implementation of effective support.

Interventions detailed in care plans should be based on evidence to inform an understanding of why a particular approach or action is being taken. Evidence can be applied from research, policy or practice, and used to identify appropriate courses of action in response to particular situations (Mathews & Crawford 2011). Again it will be important to apply such evidence with the recognition that results will not always be as expected, so flexibility in responding to the individual remains imperative.

Different services may have 'standard' assessments and care plans that are expected to be used with all people presenting with a particular condition or who receive support from that service. While these can usefully inform some interventions (reducing risk related to pressure damage (Waterlow 2005)), and/or help ensure that all areas are addressed in others (Roper, Logan & Tierney 2000), they can encourage a narrow focus on the need rather than the individual and so should always be used with caution, ensuring that the person remains central to the support provided.

*Implications for practice*

- As with any guide for practice, care plans (and the support they 'prescribe') can become over-formulaic and result in an emphasis on the process rather than the person. Plans need to be clear

so they can be understood and implemented, but flexible to respond to the individual and to any changes.
- A person-centred approach is vital to ensure the individual remains at the centre of the support, with due attention to their goals, aspirations and what is important to them.

**FURTHER READING**


- Aveyard, H. & Sharp, P. (2009) *A beginner's guide to evidence based practice in health and social care* (Maidenhead: Open University Press).
- Hayes, S. & Llewellyn, A. (2010) *The care process: Assessment, planning, implementation and evaluation in health and social care* (Newton Abbott: Reflect Press).
- Lloyd, M. (2010) *A practical guide to care planning in health and social care* (Maidenhead: Open University Press).


## charities and third-sector agencies

SEE ALSO **employment; philosophical approaches; terminology**

The relationship between charities and people with learning disabilities is not at all straightforward. Early branding devices such as those employed by Mencap (Little Stephen) and The Spastic Society, which later became Scope (the 'crippled boy wearing a calliper and leaning on a walking stick'), reinforced the images of tragedy and pity often associated with people with learning disabilities. Recent changes to branding have resulted in more positive depictions of people with disabilities achieving change and living fulfilling lives.

Many charitable organisations were formed by parents of people with learning disabilities in response to the lack of services offered by the public and private sectors. This proactive development of services continues to the present day as local community-based groups respond to meet the needs of people with learning disabilities. Entrepreneurial individuals with learning disabilities are also developing their own charitable organisations, for example Jen Blackwell, a woman with Down syndrome, won the 'Inspirational business woman of the year' award in 2015, in an event that attracted over 600 non-disabled entrants. Her training company, DanceSyndrome, uses dance to raise awareness of learning disability issues.

In addition to providing direct services for people with learning disabilities, and training for students and staff in a range of disciplines many learning disability organisations actively campaign for improvements in rights and promote the development of public services. In some instances, they are holding local authorities, the NHS and even international organisations to account. For example:

- Bradford People First successfully campaigned for the removal of derogatory terms such as 'retard' and 'subnormal' from the World Health Organization's International Classification of Diseases (World Health Organization 1992). These terms will cease to be used when the new Classification is published in 2017.
- *Death by indifference* (Mencap 2007) highlighted the institutional discrimination of people with learning disabilities by the NHS.
- CHANGE, an organisation based in Leeds, pioneers a co-working model whereby people with learning disabilities work alongside non-learning-disabled peers to campaign for human rights developments for people with learning disabilities in the UK and several Eastern European countries.
- Shaun Webster, a project worker for CHANGE, is a tireless campaigner for the rights of people with learning disabilities in the UK and across the world. He was awarded the MBE in June 2015 for this work, one of the very few people with learning disabilities ever to receive such an award.

A web-based resource, Check the Map (see below for the link), provides contact details for a wide range of organisations across the country. These range from 'People First' self-advocacy groups run for and by people with learning disabilities, to employment support services and countryside walking groups.

*Implications for practice*

- As public services are reduced, many people with learning disabilities are using local voluntary and charitable organisations, also known as third-sector services, for support.
- Increasing numbers of social workers and learning disability nurses are seeking employment in third-sector services, which they say enables them to practice creatively and work more directly with people with learning disabilities. This is in contrast

to the assessment and review tasks which they say limit creativity in public sector services.

**FURTHER READING**

- CHANGE, www.changepeople.org.
- Check the Map, www.checkthemap.org/display?getSector_fixed=accessibility_services.

## childhood

SEE ALSO **care planning; interprofessional practice; mental health; parents; person-centred approaches; siblings**

Children with learning disabilities are children first, and for many, most aspects of their early lives will be little different from their peers. Some children have profound disabilities at birth, meaning that they and their families will need extra support to enable them to lead fulfilling lives; however, the first indication that parents may get that their child might have a developmental delay or a learning disability is that the child is not meeting developmental milestones associated with children of a similar age.

These milestones cover gross and fine motor skills, language and social development with specific indicators expected. For example by the age of nine months children would be expected to get into a seated position alone (gross motor), have an immature pincer grasp (fine motor), make talking sounds (babble) in response to others (language) and enjoy peek-a-boo (social) (Gates et al. 2015). Delays can be experienced in any, or all, of these areas of development.

Development usually happens within an identified age range, and while some slight deviation either way could be expected, early identification is important and should be discussed with a medical practitioner to determine appropriate action. Parents may not always be aware of developmental milestones, and so the role of the health visitor and other health professionals who have contact with the family is vital to ensure identification of any delays and to ensure further assessment.

Parents might need considerable support through the process of assessment which, whatever the outcome, can be an emotional and difficult experience. Parents of children with a learning disability often go through the grieving process for losing an imagined perfect baby (Raphael Leff 1991), and feelings of shame, guilt and anger are often experienced.

When making assessment, developmental age is considered to be from due date rather than actual birth date – until the child is two years old – to account for the additional developmental processes required by premature babies.

All children born with learning disabilities are considered to be 'children in need' under the Children Act 1989. While this affords them some rights, it does not automatically mean that they will be subject to legal interventions from health and social care teams.

The Sheldon Report (Florentin 1968) recommended that Community Learning Disability Teams be set up so that children with disabilities could receive coordinated and comprehensive assessments to identify need and provide treatment and therapies. More recently, the National Service Framework (NSF) for Children, Young People and Maternity Services, Standard 8 states: 'Children and young people who are disabled or who have complex health needs receive coordinated, high-quality child and family-centred services which are based on assessed needs, which promote social inclusion and, where possible, which enable them and their families to live ordinary lives' (Department of Health 2004, p. 5). The NSF notes that many children with learning disabilities will not receive a specific medical diagnosis, so predicting future needs is difficult, with each child's needs varying hugely.

Good multi-agency assessment of need is essential as the conduit for early intervention and individualised child and family focussed care packages. Despite policy recommendations supporting the value of interdisciplinary team working, there has been a decline in numbers of professionals working within multidisciplinary teams, with over one-third of all teams reporting a reduction in their funding and staffing numbers over the last five years. Over 20 years of research shows child development services and community disability team provision still varies widely across the UK for children with disabilities (Parr et al. 2013).

Many disabled children and young people have poor experiences of healthcare, social care and educational services. *Right from the start* (Council for Disabled Children 2015), identified that parents and carers can often struggle to find their way around the complex systems to get the services their child needs. Coordination of healthcare for disabled children can often involve several healthcare disciplines at primary, secondary and tertiary level. The report asserts that the quality of care that children and young people receive, and the quality of their lives, is dependent on good multidisciplinary care planning and treatment.

Of children with disabilities, 30 per cent are likely to experience poor mental health and behavioural problems, compared to 8 per cent for those without disabilities (Emerson & Hatton 2007a; Department of Health 2004). Yet this group of children are less likely to access appropriate Child and Adolescent Mental Health Services (CAMHS) than their non-disabled peers (Bernard & Turk 2009). Equality of access to CAMHS is pivotal to ensure appropriate access to diagnosis and interventions for autism spectrum conditions (ASC), attention deficit hyperactivity disorder (ADHD), conduct disorders, psychiatric disorders and challenging behaviour.

In March 2014, the Children and Families Bill was successfully passed through Parliament, becoming the Children and Families Act 2014. Part 3, the first learning disability-specific section of an Act of Parliament, places duties on local authorities, health and education in relation to both disabled children and young people and those with special educational needs (SEN). Education Heath and Care Plans (EHC Plans) replace Statutory Assessments and Statements of Educational Needs, and the framework of health, education and social care assessment is available for children and young people from the age of 0 to 25, thus supporting the transition from children's to adult services. The Children and Families Act 2014 provides the legislative framework that can help improve coordinated services for disabled children and young people to achieve the best possible outcomes in all areas of their lives. The Act states that children, young people and their families must be consulted in relation to the services available, and health and wellbeing boards should ensure strategic commissioning of services reflects those views.

This has been complemented by the Care Act 2014, which established the principle that family carers for disabled young adults must get the recognition they need. These new pieces of legislation recognise the importance of getting the interaction between different services in disabled children and young people's lives right, recognising the aspirations that disabled children have and listening to the views, wishes and feelings of children and their parents/carers, ensuring full participation in all decision-making.

*Implications for practice*

- Any parental concerns regarding delayed development of their child should be taken seriously and certainly never dismissed.
- It is important to observe the child and take a full account of parental concerns to further inform assessment.
- Referral to a paediatrician should be made as soon as possible where concerns persist, or where regression from a previously acquired skill is noted.
- It is important not to offer false reassurance to parents but to provide clear and factual information based on the individual situation of the child.
- Local authorities and healthcare providers use the Register of Disabled Children and Young People (proposed by the Children Act 1989) to assist in planning service provision, including short break services. Parents should be encouraged to consider registering their child's details to assist in demographic planning.

**FURTHER READING**

- Child development information, www.nhs.uk/Tools/Pages/birthtofive.aspx.
- Children and Families Act 2014 (London: The Stationery Office).

## communication

SEE ALSO **assistive technology; behavioural approaches; discrimination; ethnicity; healthcare services**

One of the biggest barriers that people with learning disabilities face in leading an 'ordinary lifestyle' with full access to rights and community participation is communication (Joint Committee on Human Rights 2008). It is estimated that 50–90 per cent of people with learning disabilities have some form of communication difficulty (Jones 2002), meaning they may have some barrier to making their needs known, expressing their choice and wishes, and engaging in social interaction.

It is important to recognise that just because somebody does not use words, this does not mean that they are unable to communicate. It is suggested that in general communication, only a small percentage of the message is conveyed in the words, with the rest being unspoken factors such as gesture, body language, facial expression and tone of voice. This knowledge opens the opportunity for us to understand communication in a different way which we can begin to relate to people who do not use words in the traditional sense of language and communication. This can apply to both receptive communication (what a person understands about what is being said to them) and expressive communication (what a person is trying to say to others).

Many individuals who do not use words try to communicate their needs, choices, likes, dislikes, feelings etc. in a range and combination of different ways including vocalisations, gestures and behaviours. Over time this can be developed into a personal communication system as individuals work with those around them to interpret and understand these actions. In some cases, this can be documented on a communication chart (Helen Sanderson Associates 2016a) which identifies the context of a particular action occurring, what this might mean the individual is communicating and, importantly, what the response to this should be. For example at any time of the day David may put his hand down his trousers, we think this means he needs to go to the toilet and so he should be supported to the bathroom. In a similar process, this can be reversed to detail how to more effectively communicate with the individual by identifying what we want the person to do, how we communicate this to them and, importantly, what support they might need to do this. These charts can be developed into 'dictionaries' that can be used to support individuals more effectively.

Some individuals may use other means in order to enhance communication, such as signs, pictures, photographs, drawings, real objects etc., and these can be used in a very personal and individual way, as above, or within the framework of a more formal system requiring some level of knowledge and/or training. These methods of communication are referred to as augmentative and alternative communication systems (AACs) which support, or replace, traditional communication such as speech and writing.

Sign language is a well-recognised example of alternative communication, used principally by some people in the deaf community. Other sign-based systems such as Makaton and Signalong are augmentative in that signs are used to supplement speech by emphasising key words to aid understanding.

Pictures and symbols can be used in a similar way to emphasise the key points of a communication, or for a person to point to in order to express choices. Frameworks such as the picture exchange communication system (PECS), talking mats or picture boards can be used with pre-existing images and formats that can be personalised depending on individual needs.

For some people, objects of reference are a helpful way of enhancing communication through an association of specific objects to particular meaning, whether that be a person, activity or a more abstract concept such as an activity coming to an end. Sounds and music can be used in the same way.

Accessible information is a term used to describe methods of making written documents more understandable for people who can't read or may not understand the complex way important documents are written. This usually involves the use of symbols and pictures, such as with Easy Read or Widgit, alongside more straightforward written explanations. The importance of providing information that is easier to understand is highlighted by the government's implementation of an Accessible Information Standard (NHS England 2015) that details a phased approach to ensure that by July 2016, all organisations providing NHS or publicly funded adult social care must fully comply with the standard's requirements for accessible information.

The development of technologies in the last ten years has made electronic forms of communication far more accessible than might previously have been the case, and there are a range of apps that can support individuals using pictures and symbols, and can 'translate' these into spoken words.

Many people have developed ways of recording their preferred methods of communication in order for people they meet in different settings to be able to communicate more effectively with them. These may be quite general in the form of a Communication Passport, or they might have a specific purpose and include key information to support the individual in a particular setting, such as medical information in a Hospital Passport.

As well as the practical aspects of communication in making needs known and meeting them, social communication helps build relationships and reduce exclusion and isolation. Physical barriers with communication can be exacerbated by a lack of understanding of social rules, processing difficulties that mean conversations can be difficult to follow, and anxiety because of previous negative experiences. Social communication can be hard when working with people with profound learning and communication disabilities. Intensive Interaction is an approach that has developed as a way of creating enjoyable interactions and learning together the fundamentals of communication, based on the expression of the individual.

Improving communication support for people with learning disabilities has been high on the agenda in government policy, reports and guidance over the last 15 years, with *Valuing People* (Department of Health 2001) and the update *Valuing People Now* (Department of Health 2009a) emphasising the importance of ensuring that people who support those with a learning disability listen to them and adapt their own communication strategies in order to understand what people are expressing.

It will also be important to consider ethnicity and culture and how these may impact on communication styles as well as if English is someone's first language. It will be important to ensure that as a practitioner you have sufficient knowledge and understanding of an individual's ethnicity, culture and language when communicating with them.

This attitude of adapting and taking the time to understand how and what people with learning disabilities are communicating is vital in supporting individuals. All people try to communicate, but their communication methods are often not understood by those around them, and it is up to those people to use a range of different skills and whatever actions or tools are available to them to ensure they learn from experience and better understand and support the individuals they are communicating with. It is also the responsibility of services to make reasonable adjustments that account for AACs both in written and verbal communications, to ensure information can be understood.

Whatever the communication method, consideration should be made to having a helpful environment, free from distractions and comfortable for the person to express themselves. Good communication will let the person lead and be at their pace, giving them time to respond, as it may take them a little longer to process information than might be expected. Communication should be clear, with simple language, checking back understanding and giving feedback to develop better communication in future. Knowing the person and their communication approach is vital, but there are times when understanding can be enhanced by working with someone who knows the individual well and can help support and interpret communication.

It is vital to remember that all individuals will use and respond to different communication methods in different ways. Some people will not link abstract pencil drawings and symbols to actual objects, places or choices, and so physical objects or photographs may be better for them. Introducing new communication tools can also take time, as individuals will need to develop understandings and associations, for example with any symbols or objects used.

Every individual is different, and working in a person-centred way to learn, develop and share effective communication will enhance the choice and control they have over their lives and empower them to remove barriers and have greater participation and inclusion.

*Implications for practice*

- When working with people with learning disabilities, it is important to display positive values; this includes working from the premise that everyone can communicate, but they may do this in ways which others may find hard to understand.
- The onus is on people around the individual to learn and adapt to their communication strategy and to work together for better understanding.
- There are a range of tools and systems of communication that can help support communication, but each individual will have their own preferences and it may require patience and creativity to find effective ways of developing communication with people.
- If a person has their own method of communicating certain things, then it is vital to document and share what and how they do this so that everyone who is close to that person knows and understands what support is required.

**FURTHER READING**

- Goodwin, M., Edwards, C. & Miller, J. (2015) *Communicate with me: A resource to enable effective communication and involvement with people who have a learning disability* (London: Speechmark).
- British Sign Language, www.british-sign.co.uk.
- Communication Boards, www.amyspeechlanguagetherapy.com/communication-boards.html.
- Communication Passport, www.communicationpassports.org.uk/Home/.
- Easy Read, www.changepeople.org.
- Hospital Passport, www.nhs.uk/Livewell/.Childrenwithalearningdisability/Pages/Going-into-hospital-with-learning-disability.aspx.
- Intensive Interaction, www.intensiveinteraction.co.uk/.
- Objects of Reference, www.communicationmatters.org.uk/page/using-objects-of-reference.
- PECS, www.pecs-unitedkingdom.com.
- Signalong: The Communication Charity, www.signalong.org.uk.
- Talking Mats: www.talkingmats.com.
- The Makaton Charity, www.makaton.org.
- Widgit, www.widgit.com/.

The examples of AACs given above do not reflect all the different systems that are available for use, or indicate an endorsement of them over other systems.

## criminal justice and forensic services

SEE ALSO **joint enterprise and mate crime; radicalisation**

Tensions between care and control are central to the debate of how to support people with learning disabilities who commit crimes. People with learning disabilities have been portrayed as biddable individuals, easily persuaded into joining gangs or committing crimes at the behest of others. This view suggests that they are in need of care and support (Clark 1894; Banham Bridges 1927), but they have also been portrayed as a threat to morality and purity, requiring euthanasia or at least permanent incarceration in rural locations where they could not 'contaminate' the rest of society (Tredgold 1909).

Research into criminal activities and people with learning disabilities is not new, yet we still know little about how to effectively support vulnerable people in or around areas of criminal behaviour and justice. Recent findings indicate that low intelligence, poverty and mental ill health are all significantly connected to a person embarking on a criminal activity. Unsurprisingly, people with learning disabilities are less likely to cover up their crimes, less likely to remember the consequences of their actions and are thus more likely to repeat them and be repeatedly caught. They are more likely to confess, including making false confessions, and less likely to understand the criminal justice system (Banham Bridges 1927; Emerson & Hatton 2007b; Talbot 2008).

Approximately a quarter of children and young people in the youth justice system have learning disabilities (IQ <70), with a further third having borderline learning difficulties (IQ 70–80). A response to this has been the development of forensic child and adolescent mental health services, which began to emerge around 2009. These multi-professional teams aim to help the child and their family to recognise destructive patterns of behaviour, develop self-protection skills and thus prevent reoffending.

While many children and young people are now being successfully diverted from the criminal justice system (CJS), and are therefore never convicted of a crime, there is limited evidence of effective intervention that prevents reoffending, as many continue to present 'offending-like behaviour' in adulthood. This group of people tend to be admitted as patients to specialist forensic hospitals, more commonly known as 'secure units'. There are approximately 1356 low-security, 414 medium-security and 48 high-security beds in England, costing around £300 million a year, yet there is scant empirical research into the effective management and support of this group, as identified by the Mental Health Research Network – Clinical Research Group Forensic Intellectual and Developmental Disabilities (2015).

It is suggested that 20–30 per cent of all offenders in UK prisons have a learning difficulty or disability. Further research suggests that 7 per cent of adult offenders have a learning disability, with a further 25 per cent having an IQ <80 (Department of Health 2011a). Several reports have highlighted that there is a generally poor understanding of the issues facing people with learning disabilities in the CJS. In particular, staff commonly do not recognise when an offender has a learning disability, do not support them effectively while in custody and tend not to involve other services in assessment and discharge (Lord Bradley 2009; Loucks 2007; Talbot 2008; Talbot 2012).

It is important to note that the CJS does not currently distinguish between offenders with learning disabilities and learning difficulties, the two conditions being conflated and referred to as LDD. Attempts to improve this situation have been made, notably through the publication of a handbook for CJS staff (Department of Health 2011a); however, lack of recognition has a significant impact on the likelihood of people with learning disabilities completing programmes designed to assist offenders in understanding their crimes and preparing them for release. For example the Thinking Skills Programme (Ministry of Justice 2008) aimed at reducing reoffending was only available to people with an IQ over 80, which effectively prevented people with learning disabilities from accessing the training. Further work by the Foundation for People with Learning Disabilities (2014a) has been done to adapt this for people with learning disabilities.

A joint inspection of the treatment of offenders with learning disabilities within the criminal justice system, undertaken in 2014, revealed that 30 per cent of offenders fall into the category of LDD (HM Inspectorate of Probation et al. 2014). The report noted the ongoing lack of learning disability training for custody sergeants and force medical examiners, and a general lack of understanding by police officers of the difference between mental health and mental capacity. The inspection report recommended that all CJS agencies adopt a definition of learning disability and develop an effective screening tool available in all custody suites. At the time of writing, the Learning Disability Screening Questionnaire (McKenzie & Paxton 2005) consists of seven questions and need not be delivered by a qualified learning disability professional. The report also recommended that alleged offenders should have access to trained, good-quality appropriate adults (responsible for protecting rights and welfare) in and out of hours and that custody suites should contain areas which provide privacy for detainees during the initial screening and booking. The easy-read guide *Staying positive* (Department of Health 2011b) was produced in response to some of these concerns. The document aims to inform people with LDD about basic procedures in the CJS from arrest through to caution, release or court attendance.

Once convicted of an offence, a person with a learning disability may receive one of a range of disposals, including community orders, restorative justice, probation orders, resettlement to specialised learning disability assessment and treatment units, or a custodial sentence. If the offence is considered serious and therefore punishable under the Criminal Justice Act 2003, the court may consider converting a sentence to section 37 of the Mental Health Act 1983, which usually entails compulsory admission to a secure psychiatric hospital. A person with learning disability cannot be considered to be suffering from a mental disorder for the purpose of imposing a hospital order unless the disability is associated with abnormally aggressive or seriously irresponsible conduct (Mental Health Act 1983; Mental Health Act 2007).

This issue of co-morbidity of mental health and learning disabilities is particularly challenging in terms of support and control following an offence, resulting in some confusion, with assessment and treatment units and forensic service beds being misunderstood as referring to the same provision. Of forensic (category 1) beds, 70 per cent are in low-security provision, which means that many people could be 'stepped down' to less-restrictive category 4 or 5 rehabilitation beds in the community (Royal College of Psychiatrists 2013). These beds would usually be overseen by specialist community services. Such services are able to support people through rehabilitation using a variety of tools which recognise ongoing support needs and triggers that may indicate that a person might be in danger of relapsing into offending behaviour. While such community options must be welcomed as enabling a person to integrate back into ordinary community life, it must be remembered that the key to success is that they must be supported by specialist learning disability forensic practitioners. Some evidence suggests that services that pursue an 'inclusion' agenda, attempting to support offenders with mental health conditions and learning disabilities in generic mental health and forensic settings, are less effective than those that provide a specialist service (Royal College of Psychiatrists 2013).

Specialist community-based forensic services provide a range of psychotherapeutic interventions, recognising that offending behaviour often has its roots in the victimisation and abuse of the offender in early life. Many offenders have complex diagnoses, including learning disabilities, mental health problems, autistic spectrum disorder or attention deficit hyperactivity disorder. Services aim to help the offender through the use of case-specific advice and support.

The most recent development in terms of community support for offenders combines the 'circles of support' model with expertise provided by criminal justice agencies to create circles of support and accountability.

*Implications for practice*

- Compared to prisoners without learning disabilities, those with learning disabilities were:
  - five times more likely to be subject to control and restraint,
  - three times more likely to spend time in segregation unit,
  - three times more likely to develop clinically significant depression and/or anxiety,
  - three times more likely to become self-injurious and/or suicidal. (National Offender Management Service 2013)

**FURTHER READING**

- Gunn, J. & Taylor, P. (2014) *Forensic psychiatry: Clinical, legal and ethical issues*, 2nd edition (Boca Raton: Taylor & Francis Group).
- *Journal of Intellectual Disabilities and Offending Behaviour*, Pier Professional/Emerald Group.
- Circles of Support and Accountability, www.circles-uk.org.uk/.

# d

## day services

SEE ALSO **employment**

Over the last decade, the personalisation agenda, influenced by the *Putting people first* concordat (Department of Health 2007), has radically changed the way in which people with learning disabilities spend their days. Prior to this, the transition from school or college to day services was reasonably straightforward, in theory. If a person was entitled to an assessment under the National Health Service and Community Care Act 1990 and found to be eligible for services, they would be offered either a place in an adult training centre (ATC) or a sheltered workshop. ATCs provided support for people who were considered to be unable to benefit from continuing academic education.

In the 1970s and early 1980s, it was not unusual for people to attend ATCs and workshops between 10am and 3pm from Monday to Friday every week; however, part-time attendance was more usual by the end of the 1990s. This was mainly due to the increasing numbers of people with moderate to severe learning disabilities surviving into adulthood and creating a greater need for services.

People with profound disabilities were often placed in day centres provided either by local authorities or health services, depending on their complexity of need. Typically, local authority centres provided support in the development of daily living skills and ongoing basic education. Many people benefitted from sessions with art, music and occupational therapists. Some centres provided soft play or 'Snoezelen' facilities to provide sensory stimulation for individuals. Health service day centres offered similar therapies and provided additional therapeutic services, supporting people with more complex health needs. Some charitable organisations provided specialist day services, for example people with learning disabilities and cerebral palsy might have been provided with specialist sessions provided by the cerebral palsy society – now known as Scope.

*Valuing Employment Now* (Department of Health 2009b) proposed employment targets for people with learning disabilities, including those with complex health needs, citing the importance of employment as a means of developing social contact and tackle poverty. *Valuing People Now* (Department of Health 2009a) had previously noted that while paid employment would be a challenge for people with complex needs and who were medically dependent, it should remain an aspiration for all. Many parents and learning disability organisations remain sceptical about the possibilities of paid employment for people with complex needs. However, the goal of meaningful activity outside the home remains an important one. 'Raising our sights' (Mansell 2010), a report into the development of more appropriate support for people with profound and multiple learning disabilities, recommended that local authorities should make meaningful educational, employment and leisure activities available on a sessional basis. It also encouraged them to make more places accessible in the ordinary settings used by non-disabled members of the community rather than confining people to specialist services for people with complex needs. The report supported the replacement of specialist day centres with person-centred activities supported by personal assistants.

The issue of replacing day centres with personal support services is a contentious one. Day centres usually provide congregated and segregated daytime support, where people with profound disabilities interact only with other similarly disabled people. They are supported by members of staff trained to support people with complex needs. This type of service can be considered to be in contravention of the principles of social role valorisation because it compounds an individual's disability by sending messages that they should be kept separate from other non-disabled people. On the other hand, day centres can provide familiarity and a place where people can meet friends. Parents often like day centre provision because it provides professional support in a safe setting, enabling parents to go to work or engage in other daily living activities.

Austerity measures imposed by central government following the 2008 UK recession have meant that many people have had their day service provision reduced. Social care services have been forced to undertake comprehensive reassessment programmes, meaning that only those people with the most complex needs are still eligible for support. Local authorities have had to reassess how and where services are located. This has led to some centres closing completely and some integrating with care centres for older people and people with physical disabilities. Between 2009 and 2012, 32 per cent of local authorities closed day services and 20 per cent of those did not report providing any alternative care or support. Of people with learning disabilities who were known to social services, 57 per cent were receiving no daytime support at all (Mencap 2012a).

Where an assessment of need indicates a need for daytime occupation, people with learning disabilities are now most likely to be offered an individual budget rather than a place in a day centre. Individual budgets can be used to employ a personal assistant (PA). PAs can assist people to access everyday activities. This can be seen as a positive step forward because it enables individuals to access ordinary community services and develop more of a community presence in accordance with ordinary life principles (see entry on ***philosophical approaches***).

However, the reality of employing PAs is complex in its own right. Not only does employing a PA provide choice and control over how a person is supported, but it makes them legally responsible for complying with employment legislation such as disability and barring service checks, sick pay etc. There are some useful guides to help people learn about choosing a personal assistant and becoming an employer; however, many families choose to use a community interest company (CIC) to manage this process for them.

*Implications for practice*

- The notion of 'day services' has changed markedly in the last decade as personal budgets have allowed people to have more choice in how and where they spend their time.
- Large numbers of people with learning disabilities are no longer being provided with any meaningful daytime occupation. This appears to be due to cuts in day services and more stringent assessment procedures.

**FURTHER READING**

- Skills for Care, 'employing personal assistants toolkit', www.employingpersonalassistants.co.uk/.
- SCIE (no date) *Community-based day activities and supports for people with learning disabilities: How we can help people to 'have a good day'*, www.scie.org.uk/publications/guides/guide16/.

## dementia

SEE ALSO **ageing**

Dementia is an overarching term used to describe a range of conditions such as Alzheimer's disease, which causes damage to the brain leading to 'symptoms of memory loss, and difficulties in thinking, problem solving and language' (Alzheimer's Society 2013). Dementia will be experienced by each individual in a different way, with symptoms dependent on the areas of the brain affected. It is a progressive condition, but the speed at which it develops and the severity of symptoms will again be very individual, with mood, behaviour and sleep often affected, and physical symptoms such as muscle weakness also becoming apparent.

The British Psychological Society (2015) indicates that rates of dementia in adults over 60 years with learning disabilities is significantly higher (13.1 per cent) when compared to the general population (1 per cent). Recognition and understanding are therefore vital aspects of support for older people with learning disabilities.

Identifying dementia in people with learning disabilities can be challenging, as the symptoms on which assessment is based may have been experienced by individuals throughout their lives and changes to skills can be subtle or not accounted for in the assessment process. Self-awareness and reporting can also be difficult alongside a lack of awareness by those close to the person who may miss signs or put them down to either their learning disability (diagnostic overshadowing) or other factors, meaning that the reporting of signs may be lacking.

National Institute for Health and Clinical Excellence (NICE) guidelines (2010) advocate referral to specialist memory services for those suspected of dementia; however, individuals with learning disabilities are often referred to specialist community learning disabilities teams who may be better able to work with individuals and their carers to understand possible changes that might indicate dementia. Where this is the case, joint working between GPs, specialist dementia services and learning disability services should be evident to ensure the most appropriate support and intervention.

Dementia is often categorised into early, middle and late stages, and while the early stages of the condition can be harder to detect in people with learning disabilities, the middle stage (where symptoms become more acute) and later stage (with increased physical health and support needs) will show similar progression to the non-learning-disabled population.

Supporting people with dementia is based on many of the principles and interventions that might be anticipated for someone with a learning disability. Based on person-centred approaches, a care plan should be developed that: enhances and promotes effective communication; maintains skills and independence; uses medication and other therapeutic interventions such as psychological strategies and reminiscence/life-story work; creates familiar environments, organised in a way the individual understands; and maintains health. All such support should be regularly reviewed to assess effectiveness and minimise any distress.

People with learning disabilities may already be accessing care and support services which provide quite high levels of support. The emphasis on maintaining care for people in their own homes for as long as possible, means that these services should be sustained, as familiarity and consistency is a key element of dementia care. Effective training in dementia to account for the changing needs of individuals should therefore be available, and services should work in partnership to ensure needs are met in the best way and environment for each individual.

*Implications for practice*

- Working with adults in older age may require extra vigilance, as some of the early signs of dementia may be masked by the person's learning disability or may be missed, as for those living more independently support networks may be limited.

- It will be important to ensure early assessment from appropriate services, which may include developing a base line of skills and functioning in order to observe any changes.
- People should be supported using person-centred principles with an emphasis on maintaining familiarity and dignity (British Psychological Society 2015).
- In line with the principles of 'Healthcare for All', people with learning disabilities should be able to access mainstream dementia assessment and support services as required.
- Joint working should be encouraged to support the individual in the most appropriate and consistent environment in order to promote and maintain skills and independence.

**FURTHER READING**

- Alzheimer's Society, www.alzheimers.org.uk/.

## discrimination

SEE ALSO **charities and voluntary agencies; hate crime; healthcare needs; healthcare services; media; models of disability; serious case reviews**

Discrimination involves the unjust treatment of individuals on the grounds of certain aspects of their identity. Discrimination is shaped by the attitudes and ideas that people have formulated about people with learning disabilities. Attitudes are very pervasive in influencing how people are treated and the expectations put on them. Attitudes are made up of what we think or are told to be 'facts', how we feel about what we are told and, finally, what we then do, how we act. Many of our attitudes are shaped and reinforced by the media, and public perceptions of learning disabilities have changed and have been challenged over time as media representation has begun to portray disabled people in more positive ways, although there is still a long way to go.

Until the 1970s, large numbers of children and adults with learning disabilities lived segregated lives, with children educated within special schools, many of which included residential accommodation. Once adults, people with learning disabilities were moved on to large-scale institutional care where it was expected they would live out the rest of their lives. People's experiences within these institutions were often degrading and abusive, and supported by an ideology that considered people with learning disabilities as less than human and as a problem that needed to be hidden and contained.

Attitudes are essentially socially constructed; the status quo is maintained by those with power within society, and societal structures such as healthcare, welfare and education reflect the dominant values and attitudes. The struggle to challenge the discrimination faced by disabled people and people with learning disabilities has been hard fought and, at times, uncomfortable for mainstream society. In the late 1980s, demonstrations by people with disabilities were held outside the BBC while Children in Need was running its annual fundraiser, the objection being that such fundraising supported the traditional charity model rather than a rights-based model.

Various pieces of legislation have tried to combat discrimination, including the Education Act 1996, Disability and Discrimination Act 1995 and, more recently, the Equality Act 2010; however, it is difficult to legislate a change in attitudes. Certainly it is evident that people with learning disabilities have become far more integrated into society over the last 20 years than they previously were. Most disabled children are educated within mainstream education, and long-stay institutions are closing. While inclusive education has been a long-cherished goal for learning disability campaigners, it has come at a price for some who are excluded from school. Reasons for exclusion include the school being unable to support behaviour which disrupts the learning environment and educational attainment being so low as to threaten the school's ranking in examination league tables.

Currently the closure of some assessment and treatment centres is also taking place. It is testament to how entrenched attitudes have been to people with learning disabilities that only now, after the Winterbourne View scandal in 2011 and the death of Connor Sparrowhawk in 2013, the government is committed to the closure of 50 per cent of such centres. This means that some people with learning disabilities will continue to be sent away to segregated assessment and treatment centres rather than benefitting from mainstream health services.

There is still widespread evidence of discrimination against people with learning disabilities in terms of employment. Some of this is due to low expectations of people with learning disabilities, and their parents being told that the person will never be able to hold down a job. However, much is due to prejudice from employers who fail to recognise the passion, commitment and skill that people with learning disabilities can bring to their workplaces. Discrimination is also rife within employment, with 21.2 per cent of people with learning disabilities reporting being physically assaulted, 44.2 per cent being verbally insulted and 56.9 per cent being shouted at in the workplace (Fevre et al. 2013).

People with learning disabilities are also discriminated against in terms of healthcare. The General Medical Council (GMC) highlighted three particular areas of concern in terms of individual and institutional treatment and care of people with learning disabilities:

1. Diagnostic overshadowing.
2. Attitudes and assumptions.
3. Institutional discrimination. (GMC 2016)

The report into Southern Healthcare NHS Foundation Trust's failure to investigate more than 1400 unexpected deaths of people with learning disabilities (Mazars 2015) provides further evidence of how the lives of people with learning disabilities continue to be devalued.

Discrimination is not limited to health and education; the criminal justice system also fails to make reasonable adjustments for prisoners and people with learning disabilities who are questioned under suspicion of having committed a crime. A consequence of this is the over-representation of people with learning disabilities in prisons and of people with learning disabilities who take their own lives while in custody.

It is important to take into account the impact of intersectionality within the lives of people with learning disabilities. Intersectionality is the understanding that oppression affects individuals in varying configurations and in varying degrees of intensity. Often people see an individual's learning disability as their primary identity and the sole aspect of discrimination they may face. People with learning disabilities may face multiple and varied discrimination, as black people, as women or because of their sexuality or any other aspects of identity that influence a person's life.

*Implications for practice*

- Part of tackling discrimination has been the recognition of the need for legislative, political, economic and attitudinal change. As practitioners, we cannot address discrimination unless we have a good understanding of the causes of discrimination alongside a knowledge of ourselves, our values and how to effectively challenge discrimination.
- Anti-oppressive practice is a core principle of social work and nursing values; it is an approach that seeks to reduce, undermine and eliminate discrimination and oppression and remove the barriers that prevent people from accessing services, and it gives us the tool to do this. Practitioners must learn how to use the tools of anti-oppressive practice.
- Working in a person-centred way is also at the heart of challenging the discrimination that people with learning disabilities face.

**FURTHER READING**


- Shakespeare, T. (2014) *Disability rights and wrongs revisited,* 2nd edition (New York: Routledge).
- Thompson, N. (2006) *Anti discriminatory practice* (London: Palgrave Macmillan).


## down syndrome

SEE ALSO **ageing; healthcare needs; healthcare services; person-centred approaches**

Down syndrome is the most common genetic cause of learning disabilities, with roughly 1 in every 1000 babies born in the UK having the condition (Morris & Alberman 2009). It is perhaps the condition most commonly associated with learning disability, due to distinctive physical characteristics that many people with Down syndrome share. While all people with Down syndrome will have some level of learning disability, it is important to remember that they are all individual with their own character, personality, strengths and needs.

Down syndrome is caused by an extra copy of chromosome 21 within the human DNA. It is not known what causes this replication, but unlike other genetic conditions it is not hereditary and appears to happen by chance in all races, cultures and social classes. Maternal age at birth is, however, known to increase the chances of Down syndrome occurring, with 1 in 1250 births when the mother is aged 25, increasing to 1 in 30 at age 45. Most commonly, people with Down syndrome will have the extra chromosome within every cell in their body (trisomy – 94 per cent), though for a minority it may only be present within some cells (mosaicism – 2 per cent) or when a piece of chromosome 21 attaches itself to other chromosomes (translocation – 4 per cent).

There are a number of physical features associated with Down syndrome, most notably facial (flat nose with small nasal bridge, eyes slanting up and out, small mouth, large tongue), but also affecting the hands (broad hands, short fingers, single palmar crease) and feet (large gap between first and second toe). It is important to recognise that not all people with Down syndrome have all these characteristics and will not all look the same. Other typical features are more systemic, with significant examples including:

- Musculoskeletal impacts (hyper flexibility, poor muscle tone, atlanto axial instability).
- Cardiovascular (abnormalities, disease).
- Respiratory (inefficient respiratory system with reduced lung capacity; exacerbated by physical characteristics which compromise airway, e.g. large tongue, small dental arch, small nasopharynx and large tonsils and adenoids).
- Gastrointestinal (bowel abnormalities, digestive issues and increased likelihood of gastrointestinal reflux disease).
- Endocrine (hypothyroidism).
- Neurological and psychiatric (learning disabilities, depression, behavioural problems, autism, ADHD, Alzheimer's in 60 per cent of people over 60).
- Haematological (reduced immune system with increased risk of infections and blood disorders).
- Sensory (visual and hearing impairments caused by structural abnormality and infection).

Such characteristics can lead to significant health implications that are evident either as a direct result of abnormalities, or as a consequence of their impacts. For example people with Down syndrome are identified as susceptible to obesity. This may be because weight control by exercise can be difficult due to reduced muscle development and strength; poor lung capacity affects stamina; and as a consequence of hypothyroidism.

Support issues may also contribute to exacerbation of health impacts, with communication difficulties and participatory barriers that are evident for many people with learning disabilities meaning that difficulties are not identified or effectively supported through preventative and/or early intervention.

There is significant evidence that people with Down syndrome may experience Alzheimer's disease at a younger age than would be expected in the general population (Thompson 2007), and so it is vital to acknowledge and recognise the early symptoms in order to provide effective intervention, including appropriate training for staff and planned care transitions if needed (Iacono et al. 2014). The entry on ***dementia*** considers this more generally.

Another factor to consider when supporting individuals with Down syndrome and their families is the impact on their emotional wellbeing from very public questions about the validity and viability of foetuses with the condition. The ability to detect the probability of Down syndrome in utero, and the decision over whether to abort the unborn child, can have devastating impacts on parents and lead to a negative concept of self through internalisation of social stigma for individuals (Saha et al. 2014).

*Implications for practice*

- As with all learning disabilities, people with Down syndrome face significant barriers to accessing society and communities as equal citizens.
- Effective support to overcome these barriers will be the primary focus of supporting individuals and families alongside treatment of some of the 'symptoms' of health complications identified above.
- These can be achieved through effective family support to ensure early intervention and promotion of learning and development throughout education, transition to adulthood and

independence, and to ensure employment opportunities are available and supported.

- Every person with Down syndrome will have their own strengths, needs and aspirations, and person-centred approaches with effective coordination or required services should be employed to ensure active participation in society.

**FURTHER READING**

- Down Syndrome Association, www.down-syndrome.org.uk.

# e

## education

SEE ALSO **employment; philosophical approaches**

The 1870 Education Act made it compulsory for all British children to be educated to an elementary standard. It was assumed that children with learning disabilities would be educated to the same basic level as other children and therefore be able to contribute to the economy. However, it soon became clear that many struggled with academic skills such as reading, writing and arithmetic. Language used to refer to people with learning disabilities has changed in intervening years, with terminology used during that time now seeming offensive to 21st-century readers. Records show that the first UK school for 'idiots' had opened in Leicester in 1822, and other schools for 'the feebleminded' followed, thus creating the beginnings of segregated education. The education of children with learning disabilities has swung between inclusion and exclusion ever since.

Subsequent Education Acts have acknowledged that children with learning disabilities learn at a different pace and many have different educational support needs to non-disabled peers. Governments have continued to respond to this by labelling children. The Education Act (1981) used the terms educationally subnormal-moderate (ESN-M) and educationally subnormal-severe (ESN-S) and recommended that affected children should be taught in specialist special educational needs (or SEN) schools. This supposedly benevolent approach sought to allow children the time and attention to develop without the pressure of having to keep up with the educational attainment of their peers. However, the reality was that much of the school day was spent developing daily living skills rather than concentrating on educational achievement. The social effect of segregation led to the isolation of children with disabilities, which continued to impact on social relationships into adulthood, with few people with learning disabilities making friendships outside the family unit. During the late 1980 and 1990s, parents and academics challenged the morality of segregating children with learning disabilities from their peers.

In 1994, UNESCO hosted a world conference on special needs education. The event took place in Salamanca, Spain. The resulting Salamanca Agreement recommended that:

- every child has a fundamental right to education, and must be given the opportunity to achieve and maintain an acceptable level of learning,
- every child has unique characteristics, interests, abilities and learning needs,
- education systems should be designed and educational programs implemented to take into account the wide diversity of these characteristics and needs,
- those with special educational needs must have access to regular schools which should accommodate them within a child centred pedagogy capable of meeting these needs. (UNESCO 1994)

The UK, a signatory to the agreement, responded by enacting the Special Educational Needs and Disability Act (SENDA) 2001. SENDA enshrined into UK law the rights of children to be educated in mainstream schools, with additional support where the latter was recommended by a 'Statement of educational need'. Schools must abide by a 'Code of Practice' (Department for Education and Skills 2002), which requires them to provide a clear statement regarding their support of special educational need. A senior manager of the school must also be designated as a Special Needs Coordinator (SENCO) and be able to influence school policy. SENCOs have a role in the assessment of a child's educational needs.

In September 2014, the coalition government announced Special Educational Needs and Disability (SEND) Reforms. These reforms mean that if a parent believes that their child has SEN, then the child has a right to be assessed. Furthermore, if the child's needs are complex, they might be eligible for an Education, Health and

Care plan (EHC). Where a parent believes their child has SEN, there are strict guidelines and timeframes during which local authorities must respond. The process is set out in the SEND guide for parents (Department for Education 2015). Assessments will typically be undertaken by a multi-professional team, including parents, doctors, educational psychologists, teachers and SENCOs if the child is already in school.

Local authorities are required to produce a Local Offer to all families in receipt of a statement of SEN or EHC. The Local Offer identifies the education, health and social care services available to children, which includes young adults up to the age of 25 years. The Local Offer must be regularly reviewed, and local authorities must respond to comments about the Offer made by parents and young people with SEN.

An early years' education system, Portage, is available for preschool children. The Portage system involves regular home visits by a Portage worker who will support the development of play, communication, relationships and learning for young children within the family. A Portage worker will also help parents to plan for their child's health, educational and social needs.

*Implications for practice*

- The integration of children with learning disabilities into mainstream schools remains controversial to date. A Mencap study of parents of children with learning disabilities revealed that 81 per cent of the 1000 parents surveyed were not fully confident that their child's mainstream educational placement was helping them to reach their full potential (Garner 2014).
- The current teacher training programme in the UK does not equip graduates with the skills to teach children with learning disabilities. Teachers wishing to specialise in teaching children with SEN must seek out local authority courses to improve their basic training. More recently, some universities have begun to offer Masters courses in inclusive education and SEN.
- Much of the day-to-day classroom support provided for children with learning disabilities is undertaken by teaching assistants, who need not have a formal teaching qualification, although they will typically have attended Local Authority SEN level 3 training, which is similar to an 'A' Level.

**FURTHER READING**

- National Portage Association, www.portage.org.uk/.
- Department for Education and Skills (2014) *Special educational needs and disability: Guidance for parents* (London: HMSO).

## employment

SEE ALSO **day services; discrimination; empowerment**

Approximately 6.6 per cent of people with learning disabilities were reported to be in some form of employment in 2010/11, yet 65 per cent say that they would like a job (Foundation for People with Learning Disabilities 2012a).

Historically, if a person had a mild learning disability and needed support to find employment, they sought the services of the Disability Reablement Officer (DRO) who was based in the local job centre. The DRO would search existing job vacancies or contact the nearest Remploy centre. School leavers might benefit from the support of a specialist transition worker from a learning disability team or a Connexions officer from the employment centre.

A second option for an individual with moderate learning disabilities was a place in a sheltered workshop funded by the local authorities. These workshops were based on production-line type skills, such as filling envelopes for mailshots, making cosmetic gift packages for high street shops etc. Each local authority would tender for contracts, which would offset the wages paid to the workers. Payment was limited to a maximum of £4 per week, so that it did not compromise any welfare benefits that the person might be receiving. The value of the workshops is debatable; people with learning disabilities often left school and moved to a workshop with their peers, and they would then spend the rest of their adult lives doing repetitive work. Parents benefitted from knowing that their adult offspring was supported during the day. Unfortunately, there was little chance of progressing from a sheltered workshop to open employment. A third strand to employment was that of 'therapeutic work' whereby a person with a disability was allowed to work for less than 16 hours per week for a token wage of no more than £28. The idea behind this was that it might encourage employers to employ people with learning disabilities on low wages. The benefits of this approach would be twofold: first, it would encourage the person to try to work without fear of losing other welfare benefits. Once established in work, they might build up their skill level and eventually be taken on as an employee with employment rights and this would offset any loss in benefits. Second, the employer would be subsidised and only have to pay a token wage while the person with the disability developed the necessary skills for the job.

Other routes into work have included the Mencap 'Pathways to employment' programme. Launched in 1975, the programme was to develop a type of apprenticeship pathway into work for people with learning disabilities. Typically a person would be referred to a pathway team, which was usually hosted by a local authority. A pathway coordinator would assess the person's readiness and interest in work and find them a job. This differed from the DRO system as it required the coordinator to contact local employers and persuade them that employing a person with a learning disability would benefit their organisation. The government provided incentives to employers, offering to pay a percentage of the worker's salary for an initial period. Coordinators might work alongside the person with learning disability or employers might provide a 'buddy' who would work with them while they developed the necessary skills to complete tasks independently. The programme was embraced by some local authorities, particularly in the North West of England.

The opening statement of this entry highlights that there is a long way to go before people with learning disabilities can claim their rightful place in employment. There has been a huge change in employment in the UK since the turn of the century, and while joblessness appears to be declining, many posts are offered with zero hours contracts that do not guarantee an income and so are unattractive for people with learning disabilities. Employers are cutting back on permanent workforce numbers, and persuading them to employ people with learning disabilities is an uphill struggle.

However, some people with learning disabilities are undeterred and have set up their own microenterprise businesses, some of which employ other people. A microenterprise is one which employs ten or fewer (full-time equivalent) people and usually has social benefit at its core. Microenterprises run by entrepreneurs with learning disabilities are still relatively rare in the UK. Typically they are supported by the family and/or personal assistant of the entrepreneur. Some have been created out of a sense of frustration by people who have gained skills during work placements but have not been successful in securing employment. Others have been created from the vision of the individual. Few microenterprises make enough profit to be viable without subsidies, leaving entrepreneurs and their families worried that welfare benefits will be taken away if the entrepreneur is assessed as having work capabilities. They are willing to take these risks due to the social benefits of the enterprise such as gaining confidence, community inclusion and status of being an employer (Reddington & Fitzsimons 2013).

The notion of people with learning disabilities as employers is not limited to microenterprises. In April 2015, Remploy became part-owned by its employees in a shared-ownership scheme. The move from government subsidy to employee ownership is indicative of the change in attitude towards the employment of people with disabilities. Congregated segregated employment settings are being replaced by open employment; however, they are still a long way away from being fully represented in the employment market.

*Implications for practice*

- It should be assumed that people with learning disabilities are capable of meaningful employment.
- Large numbers of people with learning disabilities are still working without pay, for example in voluntary services. This notion of therapeutic work should be challenged to ensure that people are paid a fair wage for tasks undertaken.
- The national living wage should apply to people with learning disabilities as it does to other citizens.
- Ideas related to co-production have also facilitated greater paid involvement of people with learning disabilities working as, for example, paid trainers of social care staff or producing accessible information.

**FURTHER READING**

- Mencap. (2012) *Stuck at home: The impact of day service cuts on people with a learning disability* (Mencap).
- CHANGE, www.changepeople.org/.

## empowerment

SEE ALSO **advocacy; assessment; discrimination; employment; person-centred approaches; sexuality**

Social workers and nurses work with some of the most vulnerable and socially marginalised people, including people with learning disabilities, many of whom experience personal or social barriers to living independently and being integrated within society. A rights-based approach and principles of social justice and inclusion are key elements in the process of empowerment and underpin all of social work and learning disability nursing practice.

Empowerment involves social workers, learning disability nurses and other professionals working alongside individuals and communities to address the challenges and barriers they face and to improve opportunities for their greater participation in society. Signposting and connecting people with local resources and supports can help develop peoples' capacity to solve their own problems.

Using models of practice based on strengths, resilience and participation, such as person-centred planning, workers focus on the capabilities of individuals, groups or communities and help them to:

- Develop the skills and confidence to express their needs and concerns, make decisions and achieve outcomes in ways that fit their circumstances and preferences.
- Have greater control and responsibility over their lives.
- Prevent the need for statutory intervention.

Much of the current legislation, such as the Equality Act 2010 and the Care Act 2014, has a focus on empowerment, with key areas of emphasis being individual budgets and direct payments. It is important to be aware of the support and infrastructure that is needed to make such ideas a success. This will involve active facilitation by workers to ensure that accessible information is readily available to ensure that people are aware of their rights. Citizen advocacy and self-advocacy groups can be useful supporting mechanisms for individuals, as they are often able to help a person to understand their issue in a wider societal context. A citizen advocacy campaign for better access to public transport is more likely to succeed than individual representation.

There are other ideas about empowerment and how to facilitate the process in practice. Peer-to-peer support is an empowering way of supporting people; peer-to-peer support means people with learning disabilities supporting each other on an equal basis and sharing common experiences. Peer support offers many benefits, for example shared identity and acceptance, increased self-confidence, the value of helping others, developing and sharing skills, improved mental health, emotional resilience and wellbeing, information and signposting, and challenging stigma and discrimination.

Co-production can also facilitate empowerment; this method of working encourages people to come together to find a shared solution to specific challenges. It involves people who use services being consulted, included and working together from the start of a project. Co-production is about human service professionals and people who use services working in equal partnerships towards shared goals. There is a movement from involvement and participation towards people who use services and carers having an equal, more meaningful and more powerful role in services. Co-production is part of a process whereby people who use services, and carers are involved in all aspects of a service – the planning, development and actual delivery of the service, power and resources are transferred from managers to people who use services and carers, and the assets of people who use services, carers and staff are valued (SCIE 2015a).

Empowerment is about fundamentally challenging and changing the power dynamics that exist between those who have power and the most vulnerable and marginalised in society.

*Implications for practice*

- The concept of empowerment links to all aspects of an individual's life and must be a fundamental value for any work undertaken with people with learning disabilities.
- Practitioners need to have a good understanding of rights-based models of disability as well as theories of power, and to aim for co-production in meeting the needs of people with learning disabilities.

**FURTHER READING**

- SCIE. (no date) 'Community-based day activities and supports for people with learning disabilities. 10 key tasks - Key task 1: Empowering people – Important things for commissioners and managers to do', www.scie.org.uk/publications/guides/guide16/tasks/empoweringpeople.asp.
- Department of Health. (2013) *Learning disabilities good practice project* (London: DH).
- Olsen, A. & Carter, C. (2016). Responding to the needs of people with learning disabilities who have been raped: co-production in action. *Tizard Learning Disability Review, 21*(1), 30–38.
- Roberts, H., Turner, S., Baines, S. & Hatton, C. (2012) *Advocacy by and for adults with learning disabilities in England: Findings from two surveys and three detailed case studies* (Improving Health and Lives, Learning Disabilities Observatory).

## end of life

SEE ALSO **loss and grief**

People with learning disabilities have stated that dealing with death (both their own and that of others) is an important aspect of their experience of growing older (Ward 2012), yet this is an issue that is not commonly addressed with people at any stage during their lives.

The experience of loss and grief for people with learning disabilities is explored in another entry, but as with other 'difficult' topics, carers and staff often struggle to discuss and support people with learning disabilities with death and bereavement, and this is especially the case when supporting individuals with profound and complex learning disabilities (Young et al. 2014).

This reticence to discuss issues of loss and grief with people with learning disabilities can equally be applied to supporting them to plan for own their own death whether that be following the diagnosis of terminal illness or condition, or as part of the process of growing older. Nevertheless, people with learning disabilities should have the opportunity for their needs and wishes to be recorded and adhered to, both in relation to any advance directives for medical treatment and also the care they would wish to receive, planning for their funeral and deciding what happens to their possessions (Ward 2012).

The need to support someone to prepare for their own death may happen in an acute way as an individual may be diagnosed with a life-threatening illness. When this is the case, intervention should follow the model set by general palliative care approaches – to improve choices in relation to care and treatment, where they want to be cared for and where they would like to die, as well as having access to high-quality care, treatment and, particularly, relief from symptoms including pain (Department of Health 2008).

Key to this is ensuring that a person with a learning disability has access to specialist palliative care services and that they can work in partnership with the individual, their carers and specialist learning disability staff in order to empower individuals to be involved in decisions about their end-of-life care (Dunkley & Sales 2014). There is evidence to suggest that this does not always happen, and just as learning disability staff are not aware of, or understand, palliative care, palliative care staff lack awareness, knowledge and confidence in supporting people with learning disabilities. A willingness to work together must be supported by more formal and strategic structures to ensure palliative care to individuals with a learning disability meets the highest standards (Ryan et al. 2010).

While staff may find palliative care situations difficult, being able to communicate and provide information to the person in an appropriate way is a key element of them being able to understand and cope with what is happening to them (Matthews, Gibson & Regnard 2010).

*Implications for practice*

- Carers and staff should have access to training and resources to help them engage with people around their end-of-life care.
- Planning for all aspects of a person's end of life and death should form part of the person-centred planning process and includes consideration of advanced directives and the making of a will within the framework of the Mental Capacity Act 2005.
- There should be a planned approach to the collaboration between palliative care, learning disability and other services with training to understand roles, processes and expectations at end of life, along with resources and guidance on how to support individuals with a learning disability during this time.

- People should be actively involved in understanding and making choices and decisions about what is happening to them, the treatment they receive and what they can expect to happen as their terminal illness progresses.

**FURTHER READING**


- Dunkley, S. & Sales, R. (2014) The challenges of providing palliative care for people with intellectual disabilities: A literature review. *International Journal of Palliative Nursing, 20*(6), 279–284.
- Matthews, D., Gibson, L. & Regnard, C. (2010) One size fits all? Palliative care for people with learning disabilities. *British Journal of Hospital Medicine, 71*(1), 40–43.


## epilepsy

SEE ALSO **care planning; discrimination; healthcare needs; healthcare services; mental capacity**

Epilepsy is a neurological condition characterised by recurrent seizures, and while there is a significant prevalence in the general population – 1 in 103 (Joint Epilepsy Council of the UK and Ireland 2011) – the incidence in people with learning disabilities is much higher, at 1 in 5 (Robertson et al. 2015). The impacts on a person with a learning disability are also likely to be more significant, and their access to treatment and support for their epilepsy may be substantially reduced when compared to the general population.

Seizures can take many forms, with over 40 potential types that are broadly categorised as 'partial' that affect only focal or localised areas of the brain, or as 'generalised' where the whole brain is affected. Partial seizures are further classified as 'simple' where consciousness is not impaired and 'complex' where there will be impairment to consciousness. Either of these can develop into a generalised seizure. Generalised seizures can be convulsive (tonic clonic) and non-convulsive (absence), and can cause significant distress to both the person experiencing it and those around them. Given the array of seizure types, it is vital for them to be recorded and relayed in terms of what is observed or experienced, to enable specialists to interpret the information and determine seizure types.

Where a seizure lasts for a prolonged period, or where there are repeated seizures with no recovery between, an individual may need 'rescue' medication as they are in 'status'. Historically this would be the muscle relaxant diazepam given rectally, but more recently midazolam administered to the buccal area of the mouth (between the gums and the cheek) is being used as a more dignified and practical alternative. While the recognised duration of where a seizure becomes status is considered to be 30 minutes, this needs to be understood in terms of the usual seizure pattern of the individual, and any change would need to be responded to appropriately. This should be detailed in a seizure management plan.

The causes of epilepsy can vary from inherited genetic factors to damage resulting from trauma. Where the cause of the condition is known, this is referred to as 'symptomatic' epilepsy. However, for the majority of people, causation is not likely to be identified ('ideopathic' epilepsy), and this figure is reflected in the population of people with learning disabilities. Specific syndromes are associated with learning disabilities where epilepsy would be described as part of the condition (Rett syndrome), and others where it would be said that it resulted from the condition, such as tuberous sclerosis where lesions within the brain cause the misfiring of signals, resulting in seizures.

While the cause of epilepsy is unknown in most cases, individuals often have triggers or sets of circumstances where a seizure is more likely to occur. These can include: fatigue; stress; anxiety; hormonal changes; high temperature; and exposure to drugs or alcohol. It should be noted that only around 3 per cent of people with epilepsy have seizures triggered by flashing lights (photosensitivity) (Joint Epilepsy Council of the UK and Ireland 2011).

It is estimated that with effective treatment 70 per cent of the population with epilepsy could be seizure-free, but the actual number where this is achieved falls below this, at just over 50 per cent. This results from delays in identification and treatment, misrecognition and misdiagnosis as well as individual responses to diagnosis and people's engagement with the treatment process. Again, all these factors increase when the person has a learning disability.

Having poorly controlled seizures can have a significant impact on a person's quality of life and the ability to access employment and other community activities, as well as reducing their life expectancy, with over 1000 epilepsy-related deaths per year – over

40 per cent of which are deemed preventable. Of the epilepsy-related deaths that occur, half are likely to be unexplained and fall within the definition of sudden unexpected death in epilepsy.

Epilepsy is most commonly treated by anti-epileptic drugs such as sodium valproate (Epilim) or lamotrigine (Lamictal), but there are other recognised treatments, including implantation of a vagus nerve stimulator (implanted electrical stimulator (Epilepsy Action 2013)) and surgery. Treatment options for children include following a ketogenic diet (high fat, low carbohydrates and controlled protein). There are clear guidelines for implementing treatment regimens (National Institute for Health and Clinical Excellence 2012), and these should be followed in consultation with specialist staff.

With the difficulties in reducing seizures for people with learning disabilities, there should be a strong emphasis on the effective management of their condition, both in reducing identified triggers for seizures and in supporting the individual effectively when they have a seizure. This process should fundamentally involve education and support for the individual to understand their seizures, and to be involved in self-management through a person-centred health action plan. People with a learning disability and their carers should have access to specialist support and advice in order to do this, and individuals should have clear epilepsy care plans and seizure management plans to ensure their health and safety and minimise risks (National Institute for Health and Clinical Excellence 2012). These would include steps to reduce the likelihood of seizures, such as medication compliance, as well as the recognition of when a seizure is likely to occur and action to be taken during and afterwards, with clear identification of the usual pattern of seizures and when to take urgent action. As with all medical treatment, care plans should incorporate consideration of the Mental Capacity Act 2005.

When an individual has a learning disability, it may be harder to recognise seizure activity, and the self-reporting of possible signs can be more complex. The greater the degree of learning disability, the more likely the individual will be to have epilepsy, and individuals may struggle to understand, interpret and communicate their experiences, as well as to adhere to treatment regimens and report their efficacy. Recognition then relies on the (paid or unpaid) carers of people with learning disabilities who may have limited knowledge of epilepsy and seizure identification and may confuse or interpret this as the individual's usual patterns of behaviour, attempts to communicate or as a behavioural disturbance. Epilepsy awareness and training is therefore vital for people who support individuals with a learning disability.

It is widely recognised that people with epilepsy experience discrimination and negative attitudes. The stigma they feel has the potential to significantly impact on some people's lives, with fear and anxiety not just of having seizures but of the reactions of others to them, leading to loneliness and them not fully engaging as citizens in their communities (Morrell 2002). A key area where this is noted is employment, where attitudes of employers to employing people with epilepsy are proven to be negative (Jacoby, Gorry & Baker 2005). This of course also applies to people with learning disabilities but it is also important to recognise that side effects of some medications prescribed for epilepsy, such as tremors or drowsiness, can affect participation or make individuals 'stand out' and actually add to isolation, discrimination and stigma. As with seizures, side effects can also be harder to identify in people with learning disabilities.

*Implications for practice*

- Recognition and recording of seizures is vital to ensure early identification, diagnosis, treatment and support.
- A person diagnosed with epilepsy should have their own recorded treatment plan and seizure management plan.
- Treatment and intervention plans should be reviewed regularly in partnership between the individual, the people supporting them and a specialist medical practitioner.

**FURTHER READING**

- Epilepsy Action, www.epilepsy.org.uk.
- National Institute for Health and Clinical Excellence. (2012) *The epilepsies: The diagnosis and management of the epilepsies in adults and children in primary and secondary care [CG137]* (London: NICE).
- *Seizure: European Journal of Epilepsy*. Elsevier.

## ethnicity

SEE ALSO **discrimination; international perspectives**

The Equality Act 2010 brought together all previous legislation that covered discrimination. The Act identifies groups of people in society who face discrimination and sets out expectations of public bodies to combat discrimination. Race, ethnicity and religion are included within the remit of the act, thereby placing a duty on local authorities to meet the needs of black and minority ethnic people with learning disabilities and their families.

*Valuing People Now* (Department of Health 2009a) identified that people with learning difficulties from black and minority ethnic groups and newly arrived communities and their families often face what is called 'double discrimination'. They experience insufficient and inappropriate services. This may be caused by:

- Policy and services which are not always culturally sensitive.
- Wrong assumptions about what certain ethnic groups value.
- Language barriers.
- Discrimination.

As a follow-up to *Valuing People*, the Department of Health, in conjunction with the Valuing People Support Team, published *Learning disabilities and ethnicity: A framework for action* (Department of Health 2004), later updated by the Foundation for People with Learning Disabilities (2012b). The key issues that were highlighted were underpinned by the need to collect accurate information relating to ethnicity and people with learning disabilities, to respond to particular needs in a culturally sensitive way and to engage with communities; the report focussed on housing, health and employment.

The UK population is diverse in terms of ethnicity, culture, language and religion; indeed, there may be a complex mix within one family. Ethnicity is a fundamental component of an individual's identity, value system and filter through which they understand the world. A learning disability is understood in a variety of ways across cultures, with it being seen as karma within a Hindu context, that is, the cycle of reward and punishment for all deeds and thoughts as the spirit is born into another body, or within some Middle Eastern cultures as a punishment from heaven, with British culture moving away from ideas of sin and punishment to the medical model of disability as recently as the 19th century and latterly moving towards the social model of disability rather than spiritual explanations.

How a disability is understood will have a profound impact on the take-up and usefulness of services offered. A study by Fatimilehin and Nadirshaw (1994) identified significant differences in the beliefs and attitudes of Asian families and white British families towards children with a learning disability. Asian families reported having more contact with a holy person for support, less awareness of medical labels and explanations of disability, and wanting care to be provided by a relative when they were no longer able to. By contrast, most white British families received a medical explanation, were not offered a spiritual explanation for their child's disability and most wanted their child to be cared for in the community in a home provided by the statutory or voluntary sector in the event of them no longer being able to care for their child. There is the potential for stereotyping and making assumptions based on ethnicity, with there being a commonly held view that Asian people do not want certain types of services for cultural reasons when, in fact, they would take up services where they are culturally appropriate.

The prevalence of learning disabilities within South Asian communities is three times higher than in the majority communities, with 19 per cent of these families having more than one member with a learning disability (Mir et al. 2001). This higher prevalence has been linked to health inequalities, high levels of material and social deprivation, and a greater prevalence of marriage between first cousins (Jaber, Halpem & Shohat 2000).

In order to work effectively with people with learning disabilities from all cultures, it is important to understand the potential impact of racism on people's lives on a personal, cultural and structural level. Discrimination will be likely to impact on education, employment, housing and healthcare, which can lead to social isolation and culturally inappropriate forms of care and service provision. It is important to understand that discrimination may permeate people's lives in a multitude of ways that will have aspects that are unique to themselves as well as aspects that may be shared with a wider community.

Cultural competence refers to the ability to work effectively with individuals from different cultural and ethnic backgrounds, or in settings where several cultures coexist. It includes the ability to understand the language, culture and behaviours of other individuals and groups, and to make appropriate recommendations. Individuals that provide services need to understand the significance of religious beliefs and cultural practices which may impact on diet, appearance, personal care, preferences for activities, gender of staff and communication (Guzman 2014). Cultural competence is not simply understanding a set of 'facts' about another culture but understanding the values, history and experiences of people, including the impact of discrimination on them and ways in which this may be countered.

The use of language can create significant barriers, with potential ambiguity on both sides that what is being communicated has been thoroughly understood. This can also happen where there is a high degree of fluency but cultural nuances may still be lost. Using interpreters is very important as they can act as the link both linguistically and culturally to people with learning disabilities and their families (O'Hara 2003). It is good practice to discuss with interpreters prior to a meeting how joint working will be carried out and to clarify the boundaries of their role, as they might be used as advocates or cultural consultants when this is not within their remit. It is important to not make assumptions about cultural practices but to work in a person-centred way that ensures individual needs are met.

*Implications for practice*

- Cultural competence needs to take into account an understanding of racism and discrimination and its impact on people with learning disabilities and their families, as well as an understanding of the values, beliefs and culture of black, ethnic minority and newly arrived groups.
- Practitioners need to ensure they are aware of the different ethnicities in their local area and know any particular health needs relating to specific groups.

## FURTHER READING


- Foundation for People with Learning Disabilities. (2012) *Learning difficulties and ethnicity: Updating a framework for action*, www.learningdisabilities.org.uk/publications/learning-disabilities-and-ethnicity-framework/.
- Raghavan, R. (2011) Commentary on 'A qualitative exploration of the life experiences of adults diagnosed with mild learning disabilities from minority ethnic communities'. *Tizard Learning Disability Review, 16*(5), 14–17.

# f

## fragile X syndrome (FXS)

SEE ALSO **autism**

FXS is the most common inherited cause of learning disability; usually 1 in 4000 males and 1 in 8000 females of the general population are affected (Contact a Family 2013). FXS derives its name from the 'fragile' gene on the X chromosome (FMR-1) that causes the syndrome.

Due to the fact that women have two x chromosomes, female carriers of the gene may be unaware that they carry it and might not have a learning disability. However, they will most often experience extreme shyness and other aspects of social awkwardness. If one family member is diagnosed with FXS, other family members should be encouraged to seek genetic testing. Early diagnosis followed by additional support in education, speech and language can be effective in helping individuals to attain more confidence and improve daily living skills.

Levels of learning disability experienced by individuals with FXS vary greatly. Some children with FXS may develop attentional, emotional and behavioural difficulties. Speech and language difficulties, including cluttered sentences, echolalia and the lack of contextual understanding, are common. Social anxiety, particularly extreme shyness and avoidance of making eye contact, are also common in people with FXS. Some individuals display repetitive behaviour, prefer a daily routine and can find it hard to adapt to change; these social and communication difficulties accompanied with ritualistic behaviours can lead to a minority of individuals receiving the label of autism (Turk 2008).

Individuals with FXS have common physical features; some can be recognised in early childhood, while others only manifest after puberty and into adulthood. Between the ages of 5 and 13, males with FXS usually develop macroorchidism (very large testicles).

Other features include long faces, large heads and protruding ears; it is only during and after puberty that the face becomes noticeably long (Hagerman & Hagerman 2002). Individuals with FXS can develop epilepsy in childhood or adulthood.

*Implications for practice*

- Multidisciplinary interventions can prove very effective with children with FXS. These should involve healthcare professionals such as learning disability nurses and occupational therapists, psychologists, speech and language therapists, and education professionals.
- Parents often report feelings of loneliness, loss and feelings of rejection towards their child when a diagnosis is first made. The Fragile X Society provides simple information, including newsletters, publications and research that families might find useful. They also provide a forum for support, understanding that family members may experience a range of emotions and may require additional support as their child approaches the usual life stages.
- Many people with FXS can and do lead productive lives, achieve academic success and gain employment, especially when given adequate support in early years.

**FURTHER READING**

- Fragile X Society, www.fragilex.org.uk.

# h

## hate crime

SEE ALSO **employment; joint enterprise and mate crime; mental capacity; safeguarding; serious case reviews**

People with learning disabilities live ordinary lives within their local communities. Children with learning disabilities may attend either mainstream or special schools. They may live with families, friends or other disabled people. They may be supported for some of the time or live with 24-hour support. While this move to community living means people with learning disabilities are able to have access to 'the good things in life' (Wolfensberger et al. 1996; Johnson, Walmsley & Wolfe 2010), it also means they are at risk of being exposed to discrimination and abuse from other people living in those communities (Fyson & Kitson 2007).

Children with learning disabilities are bullied by their classmates in both mainstream and special schools. Adults with learning disabilities are victims of financial, physical, verbal and sexual abuse. They are neglected, forced into marriage and experience domestic violence. Many of these incidents are dealt with under the 'safeguarding' procedures. Disablist hate crime incidents have been recorded by the police since 2011 and have increased by 5 per cent yearly, with an 8 per cent rise in 2014/15, and 2508 crimes recorded by the police in 2014/15 (Corcoran, Lader & Smith 2015). However, the figures from the Crime Survey for England and Wales appear to suggest that this is the tip of the iceberg, as they identified 70,000 disablist hate crimes recorded in the same time period (Corcoran, Lader & Smith 2015).

If these incidents involve a *reportable offence,* they are referred to the police. There is no actual offence under British law of 'disablist hate crime'; however, if the victim, their carer or the police believe the incident was motivated by the person's disability, there is the option for a sentence uplift under section 146 of the Criminal Justice Act 2003. This provision placed a duty on the court to increase the sentence if it believes the crime was motivated by the hostility towards the person because of their disability or that the victim was chosen because of their *vulnerability* (Crown Prosecution Service 2015).

Often people with learning disabilities experience years of abuse from neighbours or people they 'know'. The individual may have few friends who may protect them and may view the 'friendship' offered by the perpetrator as very important (Grundy 2011). Little is known about the reasons for disablist hate crime. We do know that it is likely to happen in both private and public spaces, in schools, on public transport, near shopping centres and in and around the victim's home. It also appears to be likely to be carried out by individuals and groups of people, and both females and males may be perpetrators.

Disablist hate crime can have fatal consequences; people such as Ray Atherton and Steven Hoskin have been subject to torture; branding; sexual assault; forced to ingest poison, weedkiller or medication. Several people have been murdered by being set on fire, forced into freezing rivers, made to jump from a railway bridge or beaten to death. Hate crime has also resulted in people taking their own lives or the lives of their loved ones. For example in 2007 Fiona Pilkington killed herself and her daughter who had a learning disability, Francecca Hardwick after years of abuse from youths in their neighbourhood.

It is claimed by campaigning organisations that the official figures for disablist hate crimes are the tip of the iceberg. For example, Mencap carried out a survey with people with learning disabilities which identified that 90 per cent of people feel afraid in their own homes and limit their daily activities to avoid areas where they may encounter harassment and abuse (Beadle-Brown et al. 2014). Barriers to reporting have been identified as difficulties with the police – people being unwilling or unable to report, the police being unaware of the disability as a motivating factor and a lack of awareness among service providers, families and people with learning disabilities. As a result, third-party reporting centres are now used to make it easier for individuals to report their incidents. In addition, recent initiatives such as Mencap's 2011 Stand by Me campaign, Hate Crime Awareness week, the Arc UK's 2013 Real Change Challenge, and the Safety Net campaign in schools have attempted to raise awareness among the police, service providers and people with learning disabilities and their carers/families.

Many serious case reviews have identified that people who are victims of hate crimes often experience the abuse over a long period and there are often missed opportunities for professionals to intervene. A coordinated approach is needed by services involved with individuals to safeguard them and offer practical help and support for individuals. However, in such cases, family or others have tried to warn the victim without success. There is a need to allow people to make bad decisions (see entry on ***mental capacity***) as well as good ones, and there is a fine line between protection and risk management. Ensuring the individual is making an informed decision is important, and it is the responsibility of the professional in these circumstances to offer support to the individual to enable them to understand the danger they may be in and which steps they can take to leave the harmful situation.

*Implications for practice*

- People with learning disabilities need to be supported to access communities safely. This can mean supporting them to understand what friendship means and how to keep themselves safe from predatory others.

**FURTHER READING**


- Quarmby, K. (2008) *Scapegoat: Why we are failing disabled people* (London: Portobello Press).


## healthcare needs

SEE ALSO **down syndrome; epilepsy; healthcare services; mental health; profound and multiple learning disabilities**

It has long been established that people with learning disabilities have greater health needs than the general population, yet these health needs are less likely to be addressed, with significant health inequalities existing between the learning disabled and general populations (Department of Health 2001).

Emerson and Baines (2010a) identify an increased prevalence of greater healthcare needs for people with learning disabilities generally, and for specific groups such as people with Down syndrome or profound and multiple learning disabilities (PMLD) across a range of conditions. These are gastrointestinal cancer; coronary heart disease; respiratory disease; mental health; dementia; epilepsy; sensory impairments; physical impairments; oral health; dysphagia; diabetes; gastrointestinal reflux disease; constipation; osteoporosis; endocrine disorders; and falls, trips and accidents.

There are a number of different reasons why people with learning disabilities might be expected to experience such greater health needs.

There may be specific health implications associated with a genetic syndrome, for example people who have Down syndrome are more likely to have heart defects and gastrointestinal deformities requiring higher levels of health support. It may also be that people who have *profound and multiple learning disabilities* have physical conditions that impact on their health status, including dysphagia or mobility issues.

People with some health conditions are more likely to experience additional health needs that directly result from the condition or from its effects, for example people with dysphagia experience repeated respiratory tract infections, dehydration or poor nutrition (Chadwick & Jolliffe 2009). Uncontrolled epilepsy can also have a significant impact on an individual's quality of life, with anxiety and depression often evident (Jackson & Turkington 2005) which can, in turn, actually impact on the likelihood of seizures.

A person's learning disability may have resulting implications for their self-care skills and health awareness, and carers' inability or neglect to perform tasks such as oral or ear care, or an assumption of capability that the individual can do this adequately, can lead to health issues in the longer term. Individuals with learning disabilities may not be able to identify and report their own health needs in the way that carers might expect, and so these needs may not be picked up on and may go untreated, causing more severe and additional complications. Communication barriers may also have a practical implication, as people may not be able to read health appointment letters or public health information, which means they may not have the information to make informed health choices.

The lifestyle and choices of a person with a learning disability may also have an impact on their general and specific health status. Reports indicate that people with learning disabilities are less likely to have a balanced diet and take suggested levels of exercise, with a resulting greater incidence of obesity (Emerson & Baines 2010a) and its associated health risk factors. While these health outcomes could be understood in terms of individual health choices, it is important to look at the influences on these for people with learning disabilities. The difficulties of communication of health messages has already been mentioned, but just as significant is the living and life options for many people in 'cared-for' environments where their choices and chances are often restricted. While people's behaviour and mental health status are covered by other entries, both these issues can greatly impact on an individual's physical health status through personal neglect, lifestyle/risk decisions or self-injurious behaviour, and the higher rates of mental health and behaviour issues contribute to the increased physical needs of people with learning disabilities.

It should be anticipated that factors affecting health inequalities more generally such as income, access to employment, environment, education, housing, and transport (as identified first in the Black Report 1980) apply to people with learning disabilities. In actual fact, people with learning disabilities are more likely to experience disadvantages in these areas and subsequently have poorer health as a result.

A further inequality experienced by people with learning disabilities in relation to both promotion of positive health and accessing appropriate healthcare is their experience of healthcare services, and a central problem within this is the assumptions made by healthcare staff about learning disabilities that lead to 'diagnostic overshadowing'. This happens when an individual's presentation or symptoms are ascribed to their learning disability rather than associated with an underlying physical or mental health issue.

All these factors contribute to an overall higher mortality rate for people with learning disabilities, with a reduced life expectancy and greater risk of early death (Emerson & Baines 2011). While this is changing, particularly for people with mild learning disabilities, it could still be expected that people with learning disabilities are likely to die sooner than the general population.

The increased health needs and health inequalities for people with learning disabilities have been recognised by successive government reports and guidance, from *Signposts for Success* (Department of Health 1998) to *Healthcare for All* (Michael 2008), and a range of measures have been implemented to improve the experience for individuals, with varying success.

Health checks have featured prominently, from the 'OK Health Check' in the early 1990s through to the 'Cardiff Protocol' recommended for use by GPs as part of a Directed Enhanced Service (DES) that would see them paid for completing annual health checks. The idea is that an individual is 'screened' for actual or potential health issues, with plans then put in place to address these that include a focus on the education of the individual and those who support them. The same was intended by the health action plans proposed by *Valuing People* (Department of Health 2001) and reinforced in the update *Valuing People Now* in 2009 (Department of Health 2009a). These were supported by a proposal for health facilitators to ensure the plans were implemented.

While health checks are recognised as being successful in identifying unmet health needs in many people (Robertson et al. 2014), they have not provided a solution for all people, and ongoing evidence reaffirms that the situation remains the same for many. This may be due to them being one-off assessments that are not reviewed at regular intervals, but may also be due to them not being implemented fully, with only half of eligible people actually having a health check appointment in the first year of the DES (Turner 2011).

While the health checks focus on the individual, there have also been recommendations for more structural changes in health and social care services to address societal inequalities and improve the health of the population generally. Within this, there is a commitment to education for: commissioners to ensure the services they pay for are designed to be inclusive of people with learning disabilities; practitioners so that the services they provide meet the needs of individuals; and inspectors of services who will assess services according to how well they achieve standards specific to learning disabilities (Department of Health 2008).

Including the views of people with learning disabilities and their families and carers is also proposed at every level to ensure their views and interests are taken into account, and it is important that this starts with their own health status and any care that they may require.

*Implications for practice*

- When supporting individuals with learning disabilities, it is important to consider their physical and mental health needs within the wider context of their care.
- Individuals should be supported to understand their own health and to make informed decisions about their lifestyle and heath choices. This will include recognition of any changes in health, what to do in the event of such changes and who/how to communicate them to.
- Where appropriate, this should be done in consultation with their families and other health and care staff to ensure that any needs are identified and addressed in a timely manner and supported effectively.

**FURTHER READING**

- Mencap, www.mencap.org.uk.
- Perry, D., Hammond, L., Marston, G., Gaskell, S. & Eva, J. (2011) *Caring for the physical and mental health of people with learning disabilities* (London: Jessica Kingsley Publishers).

## healthcare services

SEE ALSO **healthcare needs**

One of the central principles of *Valuing People* (Department of Health 2001), and many reports and recommendations both before (*Signposts for Success*, Department of Health 1998) and after (*Healthcare for All*, Michaels 2008), is that people with learning disabilities should be able to access mainstream services and expect the same care and intervention as their non-disabled peers.

Such statements have been required in response to significant evidence that this is not the case and that discrimination of people with learning disabilities in healthcare settings is widespread and well documented, with examples including:

- Lower participation in cancer screening (Turner, Giraud-Saunders & Marriott 2013).
- Poor treatment and abuse in specialist units supporting mental health and behaviour (Undercover Care 2011).
- Preventable deaths due to ignorance and indifference towards people with learning disabilities (Mencap 2007; Mencap 2012b).
- Higher number of premature and preventable deaths in the learning disabilities population when compared to the general population (Heslop et al. 2013).
- Learning disability being listed as a reason for a 'Do Not Resuscitate' order (Gayle 2015).
- Failure to investigate unexpected deaths of people with learning disabilities (Mazars 2015).

Findings of the many different reports into these and other examples of the discrimination experienced by people with learning disabilities when accessing healthcare have identified key themes and made similar recommendations to address inequalities and promote adherence to the basic human rights of people with learning disabilities in these settings. These can be grouped into staff awareness, communication and partnership working, structural issues and reasonable adjustments.

**staff awareness**

A lack of awareness of people with learning disabilities, their needs and how to offer effective support is seen as a fundamental reason why discrimination can occur on a very individual level. Ignorance can reinforce negative views and values, with fear sometimes magnifying this and leading to people being treated without the dignity and respect that would be expected. Staff training to better understand the needs of people with learning disabilities, to promote more positive values and to understand the legal framework of care provision is recommended for staff throughout health services and, in particular, as part of professional training.

Where this training is done well, it includes people with learning disabilities delivering the training as facilitators or co-producers, and promotes experiential learning rather than just theoretical, as it is only by working with people that barriers are broken down and confidence is developed.

### communication and partnership working

Ineffective communication has contributed to poor care standards for individuals as important information that would enhance treatment has not always been passed on or listened to, and this has directly affected clinical decision-making and outcomes. This has also been evident with families and carers who have had their views ignored when they are attempting to advocate for the people they support. Improved partnership working with individuals, their families and other services (including learning disability services) is vital in enhancing care and support as well as contributing to understanding and decision-making by both the practitioners and the individual about the treatment they are receiving.

One tool to improve communication and enhance partnership working is 'Hospital Passports' (Public Health England 2015a). These have been developed as a way that people with learning disabilities and those who know them well can capture key information for staff in hospital to read about how best to support them. As with One Page Profiles (Helen Sanderson Associates 2015), these should be used as the start of a conversation (not an end in themselves) to ensure the best care and treatment decisions are taken in consultation. Learning disability nurses are often well placed to facilitate partnership working; as they support individuals to access services (The Scottish Government 2012), they can use hospital passports to enhance their role in advocating for people with learning disabilities when they access general health services, to ensure their needs are known, understood and met and to promote communication between the individual, family and carers, and the medical and nursing staff.

### structural issues

Discrimination resulting from a lack of awareness is not just evident on an individual level – people with learning disabilities and their needs are also not considered in the commissioning, planning and monitoring of services. A more structural approach to identifying the learning disability population and understanding their needs is proposed so that these needs can be explicitly stated in local assessments. This will inform service design and delivery as well as the creation of standards for services to implement and be held accountable to. This will also enable a focus on identifying specific recurring needs and promoting good practice.

While some of this is data-driven, there are examples of how services are beginning to change in response to identified needs, with many hospitals around the UK now employing learning disability liaison nurses. Their job is to identify when an individual with a learning disability is admitted to hospital, and to support the staff involved in their treatment to work in partnership with the individual and their families and carers to ensure needs are considered holistically and that plans for treatment, care and discharge are effectively implemented.

**reasonable adjustments**

There has been insufficient use of reasonable adjustments to the way that services are provided, which means that there are still significant barriers to people with learning disabilities accessing healthcare services. 'Reasonable adjustments' is a legal term in the Equality Act 2010 which requires employers and providers of services to make changes to their physical premises and, importantly, to their working practices in order to make them more accessible to those with disabilities. An example might be that a GP ensures one of their patients with a learning disability who gets anxious when they are in busy areas is always given an appointment ten minutes prior to the surgery opening so they do not have to wait in the crowded reception area. Application of reasonable adjustments will of course be influenced by individual attitudes, but by commissioning authorities requiring evidence of these, and being able to share examples of good practice, there should be a better understanding and application of them (Public Health England 2015b).

While most attention on the barriers to accessing healthcare for people with learning disabilities is focussed on services, there are occasions where individuals are reluctant or refuse to attend themselves because of fear of medical treatment, or previous negative experiences. Reasonable adjustments are particularly relevant in these situations, and services can work in partnership to help relieve anxieties by supporting individuals through development of accessible information about procedures, visiting wards/areas before appointments, meeting the staff who will be there on the day etc.

Despite the attention focussed on the discrimination of people with learning disabilities in reports and recommendations going back nearly 20 years, and examples of positive practice identified, change has been slow, and good practice which should be universal is: 'very patchy and far from common. For the most part, innovation and good practice owes more to the enthusiasm of energetic individuals than to any structured and systematic engagement by health services' (Michaels 2008, p. 9).

It might be anticipated that because the above quote is from 2008 things would have improved, yet most of the reports identified at the beginning of this entry follow its publication, which indicates progress does remain slow. We should not, however, assume that all health services and staff are ineffective or discriminatory in their support of people with learning disabilities. Many services and individuals provide high standards of care with a willingness to listen and understand what it might mean to support individuals effectively, and to make changes to their usual working practices in order to meet needs holistically and in partnership. The structural part of joining these up to create consistently high standards of care remains the challenge for commissioners and providers of services.

*Implications for practice*

- When supporting an individual with learning disabilities in a mainstream healthcare setting, they should be afforded the same care and treatment as would be given to anyone else.
- It may be necessary for everyone involved in their care to check and communicate if there are any needs, for example with communication or the environment, that would need closer attention and to ascertain if this will require any specific support or reasonable adjustments to be made.
- Where appropriate, additional advice and support may be required from specialist learning disabilities services with a partnership approach adopted, including the individual and their family or carers.

- Services should also work to ensure that they are designed to be flexible to meet the needs of individuals with a wide range of differences, including learning disabilities.

**FURTHER READING**

- Emerson, E. (2015) *The determinants of health inequities experienced by children with learning disabilities* (London: Public Health England).

## history

SEE ALSO **employment; philosophical approaches; terminology**

The first recorded attempt to distinguish between what we currently term mental ill health and learning disability occurred in 1325. De Praerogativa Regis sought to define different groups of people in order to deal with issues of inheritance and property ownership. This seemingly benevolent practice allowed the properties or estates of people who were considered to be unfit to manage them to be given over to the King, in order that they be maintained until the person regained the competence to manage them. Terms such as fatuus, stultus, sot, foole natural and idiot were used to denote a person who had been 'handicapped' from birth and whose 'sanity' was not expected to improve. In such cases, the family estate was managed by the Crown until the person produced descendants who would be able to manage the land. Note the expectation that the person would still be able to live on and work the land, and be able to marry and produce children.

Terms such as frenetics, furioses and lucida intervalla were used to signify lunatics who were expected to recover their sanity. Their property was managed in the same way as the foole natural, unless it was deemed that they would never be able to regain their sanity, in which case the property was taken by the Crown in perpetuity.

These terms remained largely unchanged until the time of the Enlightenment, when scientific thinking began to dominate Western societies. Doctors and hospitals became increasingly powerful, and terms such as feeblemindedness entered the vocabulary. Social Darwinists such as Francis Galton and Marie Stopes highlighted the deficiencies of the feebleminded, or, in today's terminology, people with learning disabilities. Galton, Stopes and another prominent woman of the time, Mary Dendy, raised concerns that allowing feebleminded people to procreate would reduce the overall intelligence of the population. They recommended that men and women with learning disabilities should be sterilised and not allowed to mix with the general population. Thus people were isolated away from ordinary communities in asylums and colonies located far away from the growing industrial towns. It is interesting to note that while most of the staff who worked in the hospitals had no formal training and qualifications, they became known as nurses almost overnight, with the National Health Service reclassifying the institutions as long-stay mental health hospitals in 1948. People with qualifications were registered as RNMD – registered nurses for the 'mentally defective', later becoming 'the mentally subnormal', then 'mentally handicapped'. Once again, learning disability was linked with mental ill health.

Successive government policies on education and healthcare sought to keep the majority of people with learning disabilities away from mainstream services; thus by the time of the closure of the long-stay hospitals, people with learning disabilities had been absent from mainstream society for the greater part of the century. This lack of community presence led to fear and mythology around people with learning disabilities. This fear gave rise to a large number of derogatory slang terms, which will not be listed here. The term mental handicap was officially used in the UK until the 1980s and 1990s. This allowed for people to understand the condition as a medical one, as befits a cohort of people who had until recently been detained in hospital under the 'treatment' of doctors and nurses.

As the social model of disability began to challenge the medical model in the 1990s, the term learning disability became increasingly common; this acknowledged that individuals had difficulty in learning and processing information. However, some considered this term to be ambiguous, especially as we began to understand more about dyslexia and other types of educational learning difficulties.

Opportunities for people with learning disabilities began to improve quickly around the turn of the 20th to 21st century.

The publication of the White Paper *Valuing People* in 2001 confirmed that people with learning disabilities had the right to independence, choice and dignity (Department of Health 2001). The paper set out objectives for local authorities to improve services for people with learning disabilities. These included highlighting their right to live in ordinary houses, to marry and have sexual relationships, and to employment, and also included recommending the closure of long-stay hospitals. The *Putting people first* concordat (Department of Health 2007) heralded the introduction of the greater personalisation of opportunities for people with learning disabilities. This was largely due to the move away from service provision to the payment of individual budgets that allowed people the opportunity to choose how and where they spent their time. The publication of *Valuing Employment Now* (Department of Health 2009b) took this further by recommending that all people with learning disabilities, including those with moderate and severe disabilities, should be in paid employment for at least 16 hours per week.

Throughout history, most people with learning disabilities have lived and worked alongside their non-disabled peers. The difference over the last century has been their large-scale incarceration, then community reintegration.

*Implications for practice*

- There are still many people with learning disabilities who have experienced institutional care and may be living with the consequences. Practitioners need to understand the potential impact of living in such settings. In 2015 we finally saw the end of large-scale hospitals housing people with learning disabilities, with the planned closure of many assessment and treatment centres.
- It can be empowering for people with learning disabilities to know and understand their histories and to be able to share an understanding of the discrimination and oppression that they have faced and still do.

**FURTHER READING**


- Race, D. (2007) *Intellectual disability: Social approaches* (Berkshire: Open University Press).

## human rights and the disability rights movement

SEE ALSO **charities and voluntary agencies; discrimination; models of disability; serious case reviews**

The disability movement has been a force for change in the UK for more than 40 years. While its origins are arguable, the creation of the Union of the Physically Impaired Against Segregation (UPIAS) in 1974 can be seen as a pivotal time in disability politics. Rights of people with disabilities had been enshrined in international law since 1948 with the United Nations' Declaration of Human Rights. However, most European governments, including the UK, adopted a welfare approach to supporting people with disabilities. UPIAS challenged the welfare approach and fought for the recognition of rights rather than the provision of welfare. The movement grew as small groups of activists with disabilities joined together to form the British Council of Disabled People, renamed the United Kingdom's Disabled People's Council in 2006. Some consider this time to have been a golden age of disability activism, and they lament the current position where disability activism appears to have become increasingly professionalised and controlled by successive government policies. This has, according to Oliver and Barnes (2006), led to the decimation of campaigning organisations controlled by people with disabilities.

This professionalisation of disability rights organisations is also discussed by Vanhala (2011), who compares the current position of leading UK charities who are run *for* people with disabilities to the situation in Canada where they are increasingly run *by* people with disabilities. Acknowledging the UK position as a state party to the UN Convention on the Rights of Persons with Disabilities (United Nations 2006), Vanhala demonstrates how organisations such as Mencap and Scope use strategic litigation to progress the rights of people with disabilities and develop case law. This approach, while effective in achieving change, is resource-intensive and beyond the capability of most small organisations. These organisations are increasingly having to compete against each other for government funding, needed for their continued existence, and have few resources left for campaigning.

The Human Rights Act 1998, enacted in the UK in 2000, applies equally to people with disabilities as it does to their non-disabled peers. While many believe these rights to be universal, it is important to note that they were not adopted across the globe. In particular, many Muslim countries believed that the declaration of rights was a Judaeo-Christian document that failed to take into account important tenets of the Islamic faith. In August of 1990, representatives of 54 Muslim countries met in Cairo and signed the Cairo Declaration on Human Rights in Islam (Organisation of the Islamic Conference 1990). While this declaration shared many of the UN rights, there were important differences, especially in respect of the rights of women and people with disabilities.

*Implications for practice*

- The Human Rights Act 1998 applies to people with learning disabilities and is supported by subsequent guidance such as the Equality Act 2010. The UK is home to people of many different faiths and cultures, and practitioners must always be mindful to challenge practices that contravene the law of the land, especially when these might contravene the rights of people with disabilities.
- A good understanding of the Human Rights Act 1998 can enable practitioners to challenge decisions where services may be risk-averse.

**FURTHER READING**

- Luke, J. & Read, J. (2003) *Disabled people and European human rights: A review of the implications of the 1998 Human Rights Act for disabled children and adults in the UK* (Bristol: Policy Press).

# i

## international perspectives

SEE ALSO **ethnicity; history; philosophical approaches; terminology**

The UK boasts a large migrant population. It is important, therefore, for learning disability practitioners to understand that they will be required to support families who may not be familiar with, or accepting of, Eurocentric ways of understanding and supporting people with learning disabilities. Differences can include a belief held in many countries including Zimbabwe and Ghana that a child is born with an impairment as a punishment to parents for sinning against God or disobeying ancestral spirits (Tafirei, Makaye & Mapetere 2013; Hervie 2013). In these places, as in some parts of South Asia, folklore and traditional remedies, sometimes termed 'witchcraft', are still used in an attempt to cure disability. Such traditions and beliefs persist after migration to the UK, so Western medicines and methods of support may be treated with suspicion, especially by older family members (Heer et al. 2015).

Inequalities in healthcare and education for people with learning disabilities when compared to their non-disabled peers are as common across Western countries as they are in other geographical regions. For example, the likelihood of parents being supported to take a pregnancy to full term if scans reveal foetal disability is markedly different. A comparative study of health, education and social care of people with learning disabilities in Australia, Canada, New Zealand, Norway, Sweden, the UK and the USA found that Scandinavian countries are the most likely to support such pregnancies to full term (Race 2007). While early years support is similar across all of the countries in the study, the wealth and the ability of a child's parent(s) to demand attention, impact upon the likelihood of them being offered education in a mainstream school.

Many South Asian and African countries are beginning to adopt Western healthcare methods and ideas, with some stating that inclusion in mainstream education for children with learning disabilities is available for all. Unfortunately, despite governments claiming such an ideology, school attendance remains little more than a dream for many. Families, especially those from rural communities, cannot afford to send their children to school and will prioritise the education of a non-disabled child over a child with a disability. This is by no means an issue for African and South Asian countries alone. Children with learning disabilities living in rural areas of Australia and New Zealand also have limited opportunities for schooling, and access to healthcare might also be difficult (Race 2007).

People with mild to moderate learning disabilities living in rural communities in Africa, South Asia and East Asia are likely to participate in working life because many of their communities depend largely on agricultural skills for survival. In such instances, traditional daily living and other skills are privileged above cognitive and academic skills, whereas increasing industrialisation and the privileging of further and higher education puts meaningful or paid employment beyond the reach of many people with learning disabilities in Western society. An increasingly significant barrier to employment is refugee status because in most cases it is illegal to work while seeking asylum in the UK.

In recent years there has been an increase in the numbers of people seeking asylum in the UK (SCIE 2015b). An *asylum seeker* is a person who has asked for protection but has not received a decision on their application to become a refugee, or is waiting for the outcome of an appeal. A *refugee* is an individual to whom the UK government has offered protection in accordance with the Refugee Convention 1951 (United Nations Refugee Agency 2010) and granted leave to stay.

While local authorities have a duty to assess all individuals (including refused asylum seekers) if they appear to be in need of care services, they do not have a duty to provide care unless an individual has a care need above and beyond the provision of accommodation, such as personal care or household tasks. The process of seeking asylum can be protracted in ordinary circumstances, as many people fleeing oppression, war and other tyrannies arrive without the necessary proof of disability or eligibility to stay, and many are traumatised by their experiences and may not speak English, having to rely on an interpreter to plead their case to stay. People with learning disabilities also face an added difficulty because of the lack of training in learning disabilities that is provided to staff in assessment centres. Therefore, individuals with a learning disability may go unrecognised and asylum might be refused.

*Implications for practice*

- Local authorities are prevented from routinely providing support to refused asylum seekers who are in the country illegally. However, they should assess individual claims on a case-by-case basis and apply charges for services where these are provided.
- The imposition of charges in a situation where an individual is prevented from seeking employment and is ineligible for social security benefits may lead some asylum seekers with learning disabilities into homelessness.

**FURTHER READING**

- Council for Learning Disabilities, www.council-for-learning-disabilities.org/.

## interprofessional practice

SEE ALSO **professional practice; safeguarding; serious case reviews**

People with learning disabilities can sometimes have quite complex needs that mean they require support from a range of different professionals. Physical, coordination or mobility issues might need physiotherapy input, communication or dysphagia difficulties could benefit from involvement of a speech and language therapist, or an individual's or family's circumstances may necessitate assessment and coordination of care by a social worker. Interprofessional practice is the way that these, and other professionals, work together, and with the individual and their family, to provide effective support.

Interprofessional practice is referred to in a number of different ways. 'Inter' is often replaced by 'multi'; 'professional' substituted for 'disciplinary/agency'; and 'practice' interchanged with 'approach/working'. While all of these have slightly different meanings, the principles behind their use are the same, that all those people who are involved in working and supporting an individual should collaborate to ensure that they receive the best and most appropriate care. More recent focus on 'integrated care' is based upon the same principles.

The focus of interprofessional working should be better experiences and outcomes for the individual that is being supported, and it is now commonly accepted that they should be partners in their own care and therefore interprofessional working and collaboration needs to involve and include them as an active member.

Interprofessional practice starts with good communication between all of the people involved in an individual's care, but is best achieved by going beyond this to actively collaborating to ensure the best outcomes (Pollard, Sellman & Thomas 2014). Sharing information and communicating about intervention will help avoid duplication and possibly conflicting priorities and advice, but an understanding of each other's roles, alongside active learning, support, shared decision-making and coordination, will have a far greater impact.

Multi-professional teams have often been created within specific learning disability services, or when providing community support across a geographical area. These bring together specialist learning disability practitioners across a range of professions to facilitate better ways of working together. Co-location can help more collaborative ways of working, although this is not guaranteed as it requires a commitment and investment on behalf of those involved.

Some barriers to interprofessional practice have been experienced, and these have been on structural, physical and personal levels. Service funding or design often mean that even co-located teams are working for different organisations with sometimes competing demands, priorities or restrictions on what information can be shared with others. Physical barriers might include ease of access to each other or patterns and demands of work. On an individual level, practitioners can be resistant to working more collaboratively due to a lack of confidence or protection of their own professional identities. Working to overcome such barriers is vital to enhance care and work within identified good practice and policy.

The last 20 years have seen increasing governmental support for, and direction towards, interprofessional ways of working, not just for people with learning disabilities but across health and social care more generally. This builds on previous recognition of the benefits of collaboration for service users and their families, and has become an explicit theme of all major health and social care policy initiatives (Tope & Thomas 2007). It continues to underpin and support practice on an individual basis through personalisation (NHS Confederation 2015), and through structural change such as devolved health and social care budgets (Healthier Together 2014).

*Implications for practice*

- When more than one service or practitioner is involved in supporting an individual with a learning disability, they should work together to ensure that needs are met in the most appropriate way.
- Collaborative working should include and involve the individual and their families.

**FURTHER READING**


- Hammick, M., Freeth, D., Copperman, J. & Goodsman, D. (2009) *Being interprofessional* (Cambridge: Polity Press).
- Thomas, J., Pollard, K. & Sellman, D. (Eds.). (2014) *Interprofessional working in health and social care: Professional perspectives*, 2nd edition (Basingstoke: Palgrave Macmillan).

# j

## joint enterprise and mate crime

SEE ALSO **criminal justice; history; serious case reviews; terminology**

The issue of people with learning disabilities being coerced into criminal activities continues to challenge parents, carers and policymakers. If an individual joins with another person or gang with the intention of committing a crime, this is known as the 'doctrine of joint enterprise'. Under joint enterprise an individual can be found guilty if they are present when a crime is committed by another person. Perhaps the highest profile case of joint enterprise associated with a person with learning disabilities is that of 19-year-old Derek Bentley. Bentley was hanged in 1953 for the murder of a police officer during a bungled robbery, even though the offence was committed by his accomplice, Christopher Craig, who although only 16 years old, was determined to have been the instigator of the robbery and to have encouraged Bentley to participate in the crime.

Today we recognise this kind of influence as mate crime. Many people with learning disabilities lack genuine friendships and may therefore be vulnerable to mate crime. Mate crime occurs where a person befriends a vulnerable person in order to exploit or abuse them in some way (Grundy 2011). This might include stealing money, physical or sexual assault or otherwise enticing the person to engage in illegal activities.

Mate crime has been recognised as a problem since the tragic deaths of Ray Atherton and Steven Hoskin. Both men had learning disabilities and lived in their own homes rather than supported living. They were 'befriended' and subsequently tortured to death in separate incidents. The incidents were subjects of serious case reviews and were influential in the development of the Safety Net project, funded by the NHS. Safety Net was launched in two pilot areas, Devon and Calderdale, and involved joint working between the police, community leaders and local partnership boards, and resulted in the development of a training programme. The programme includes awareness training for agencies involved in supporting vulnerable adults and an easy-read booklet that aims to help people with learning disabilities to recognise the difference between 'Friend or Fake'.

Friendship is an important aspect of life; friendships help us feel part of a community and help reduce isolation. Good friendships help us maintain a sense of wellbeing. People with learning disabilities may need support to recognise true friendships and to avoid potentially destructive ones. Many people with learning disabilities choose to live without the support of services; however, it is important that they are prepared to meet the challenge of independence. People may need support to recognise how to keep themselves safe from those who might seek to befriend them in order to abuse them.

Circles of support may offer safeguards in this respect by encouraging the person to introduce new friends to existing friends in their circle. Friends should be aware of behavioural changes in the person with a learning disability, such as withdrawal from previous friendships, visiting new places – especially those that are in previously unfamiliar parts of town, the sudden appearance of new possessions (e.g. computer games, clothes) – especially when the person is reluctant to say where the new possessions came from, or increased use of alcohol or non-prescription drugs.

*Implications for practice*

- In February 2016 the Supreme Court ruled that joint enterprise had been misinterpreted in law for the last 30 years, leaving many verdicts unsafe and giving fresh hope to many people with learning disabilities who have been wrongly convicted.

**FURTHER READING**


- Bridges, L. (2013) The case against joint enterprise. *Race & Class*, 54(4), 33–42.
- NHS Safety Net, 'Friend or fake', http://arcuk.org.uk/safetynet/.

## joint health and social care self-assessment framework

SEE ALSO **accommodation; healthcare needs**

Local authorities social care services and NHS clinical commissioning groups are required to work together to improve the health and wellbeing of people with learning disabilities. Recent high profile cases have shown that despite policy papers such as *Putting People First* (Department of Health 2007), *Valuing People Now* (Department of Health 2009a) and the Health and Social Care Act 2012, people with learning disabilities are still being poorly supported by these organisations.

The Joint Health and Social Care Self-Assessment Framework (SAF) is designed to help each local authority partnership board to assess their progress in three key areas of practice.

The SAF requires each partnership board to provide information about the overall number of people with learning disabilities in their area, the number with complex or profound learning disabilities, and the number with learning disabilities and autism.

Each area or theme has a number of indicators that partnership boards are required to rate themselves against using a red, amber, green (RAG) rating system. Indicative examples of practice are given for each indicator, so that partnership boards can judge their position against the desired standard more accurately.

The themes are

- Staying healthy (nine indicators).
- Keeping safe (nine indicators).
- Living well (eight indicators).

Health themes range from annual health checks leading to updated health improvement plans, to cancer treatments, acute and specialist care and mortality. Indicators of social care support include obvious areas such as accommodation, safeguarding and employment. However, they also include the involvement of self-advocates (people with learning disabilities and carers) in recruitment and training and service planning and delivery. Importantly, a question on compassion, dignity and respect to be answered by self-advocates is also included.

Gathered data can be used by each partnership board to assess areas for local development and can also be used by Public Health England to compare data from across the country. This enables policymakers to note areas of concern, such as almost 25 per cent of people with learning disabilities living in 'seriously risky' accommodation, such as sleeping rough or in temporary homeless accommodation (Public Health England 2014, p. 99).

Another area of concern is the overall care of people with learning disabilities needing acute hospital care. Support of people with learning disabilities and autism or mental health problems (also known as co-morbidity) is an ongoing cause of concern, as is the mortality rate of people with learning disabilities, which, according to the usable data from the 2014 SAF returns, suggests that deaths of people with learning disabilities are approximately 2.1 times greater than would be normally expected in the general population. Concern over treatment and support led to the announcement of a pilot scheme in 2016. The scheme intended to provide a named social worker for every person with a learning disability and mental health problems who is at risk of hospital admission. Social workers will be encouraged to challenge decisions made about the care and treatment of individuals. It is hoped that this will contribute to the reduction of open-ended admissions to assessment and treatment units, holding clinicians to account and ensuring regular treatment reviews.

*Implications for practice*

- The joint health and social care SAF enables learning disability partnership boards to assess how well they are serving those members of their local population with learning disabilities.
- The SAF also addresses areas for development according to specified themes.
- The process is still in its infancy and has some methodological drawbacks, including data collection, which is still problematic; however, once these are resolved, the SAF returns could provide a valuable database for researchers, service planners and policymakers.

## FURTHER READING

- Glover, G., Christie, A. & Hatton, C. (2014) Access to cancer screening by people with learning disabilities in England 2012/13: Information from the Joint Health and Social Care Assessment Framework. *Tizard Learning Disability Review, 19*(4), 194–198.

# l

## loss and grief

SEE ALSO **end of life; ethnicity; spirituality**

People with learning disabilities, like all of us, experience loss in their lives. Many are the losses we all hold in common – loss of someone we love through death or separation, loss of other important or significant things like pets and familiar places, and loss of personal qualities and capacities through age and illness.

People with learning disabilities also experience losses that are unique to their situation. Valerie Sinason (2012) describes how people with learning disabilities may be affected by the grief and disappointment of their families at their birth. Parents of babies with learning disabilities experience a particular grief of their own – the loss of their dreamed-of child and the future they imagined for him or her. Health and social care professionals may encounter this grief and have to support families through it. What can be missed is the impact on the child, who feels his or her family's disappointment in them. As they mature, the child will become aware of their differences, framed as they are by the people around them as limitations, flaws or even defects. They will experience the loss associated with giving up on certain kinds of relationships, achievements and life experiences – some of which may actually be within their reach but assumed not to be by the people around them and society at large.

In addition, people with learning disabilities are likely to encounter losses as they grow up to do with being in care settings and moved around within them, losing relationships with their families, friends and care workers in the process. The common assumption that people with learning disabilities are less able to cope with change and loss can exacerbate these losses, as workers fail to include them in discussions and plans about change or offer opportunities to express their feelings afterwards. It is well understood that each new loss tends to restimulate previous losses, so that people with multiple losses, which usually includes people with learning disabilities, will be burdened with old grief as they encounter new losses. This leads to a phenomenon known as anticipatory grief, for example a person who has seen their mother die of cancer may on hearing that their father has heart disease expect his journey to death to be the same as their mother's. They anticipate the same prognosis, the same pattern of care and the same death.

People with learning disabilities are often prevented from grieving properly by these assumptions. It is common for them to be excluded from, for instance, funeral services, on the basis that they will be unable to cope, or will act inappropriately. It is sometimes even assumed that they will be unable to understand loss at all, and won't experience the feelings associated with it. Although it is possible that cognitive limitations may affect how someone understands loss, they will certainly feel the absence of a loved person or familiar place keenly nonetheless. It is also true that people with learning disabilities may, in some cases, find it harder to express their distress and need your support to do so.

It is therefore imperative that when a person with learning disabilities experiences a loss of any kind, that loss is acknowledged and their feelings validated. Basic good practice in listening and empowering clients is vital. Health and social care professionals may also need to provide creative alternatives to facilitate expression of all the feelings associated with loss and to find opportunities to process those feelings. As a basic principle of good practice, people with learning disabilities should be included in discussions, plans and events (e.g. funerals) associated with loss, with support provided to enable this as necessary.

Finally, an important factor to take into account when working on these issues is the impact on the professional helpers involved. It is well understood that emotions can be contagious and that our own losses, or fears of loss, will be activated when working on loss and bereavement with others. Practitioners need to develop awareness about their personal relationship with loss, and seek support when needed. It can be helpful to remember that although models of stages of grief abound, no one moves through them in an orderly fashion. People will move back and forth between these stages, will fail to comply with timescales and years after the event may experience a resurgence of their grief. Workers and clients alike will be affected by loss and grief uniquely, and both are entitled to opportunities to express and resolve that grief, according to their own needs and abilities.

*Implication for practice*

- It is important that when a person with learning disabilities experiences a loss of any kind, that loss is acknowledged and their feelings validated. Basic good practice in listening to and empowering people is vital.
- Practitioners may also need to provide creative alternatives to facilitate expression of all the feelings associated with loss and to find opportunities to process those feelings. As a basic principle of good practice, people with learning disabilities should be included in discussions, plans and events (e.g. funerals) associated with loss, with support provided to enable this as necessary.
- Practitioners need to understand the impact on themselves of working frequently with clients who have experienced a variety, and on occasion a multitude of losses. Practitioners need to consider their own experiences of loss and reflect on the impact on themselves It will also be important to maintain connection and empathy whilst not feeling overwhelmed. (new bullet) Practitioners who have close and intense personal contact with clients may feel burnt out and experience high stress levels. Good supervision and support from fellow team workers can eliminate some of the stress.
- People with learning disabilities can also be facilitated to set up and run their own support groups to discuss issues of loss and grief.

## FURTHER READING


- Pearce, J. (2006) 'BILD fact sheet: Loss bereavement and death' (Kidderminster: BILD).
- Scope. (no date) *Supporting people with learning disabilities coping with grief and loss* (Scope).

- Tuffrey-Wijne, I., Giatras, N., Butler, G., Cresswell, A., Manners, P. & Bernal, J. (2013) Developing guidelines for disclosure or non-disclosure of bad news around life-limiting illness and death to people with intellectual disabilities. *Journal of Applied Research in Intellectual Disabilities, 26*(3), 231–242.

# m

## maternity and parenting

SEE ALSO **human rights and disability movement; safeguarding; sexuality**

*Valuing People* (Department of Health 2001 p. 81) states that 'People with learning disabilities can be good parents and provide their children with a good start in life, but may require considerable help to do so.' Yet much of the help that parents with learning disabilities receive is as a result of reactive crisis intervention rather than supportive future planning.

A UK study of 2898 adults with learning disabilities found that 1 in 15 was a parent and that 48 per cent of those parents were not looking after their child (Emerson et al. 2005). International research supports these figures, finding that between 40 and 60 per cent of parents with learning disabilities have their children taken into care following court proceedings. These statistics provide shocking reading, all the more so when considered alongside studies indicating that there is no evidence to prove that parental learning disability equates with wilful neglect or abuse and that there is no clear link between intelligence and parenting, until IQ dips below 60 (Cleaver & Nicholson 2007, p. 14).

So why is this the case? Perhaps the answer lies somewhere in the preparation and support available for people with learning disabilities who might be thinking about having a baby. There are few resources specifically produced for women with learning disabilities who are planning to start a family; however, *My pregnancy, my choice*, produced by CHANGE (2009), is an excellent easy-read guide, approved by the UNICEF UK baby friendly initiative. The guide is part of a series of resources including *You and your baby 0–1* (CHANGE 2012) and You and your little child 1–5

(CHANGE 2013). Produced in loose-leaf binders, these publications provide essential information for keeping mother and baby well. The guides include advice on personal health, nutrition, teething, life stages and medical support. They also provide chapters about feeding a baby or child, how to communicate and play with a baby or small child, as well as developmental milestones etc.

The guide alone cannot provide all of the support necessary for a new parent, and people with learning disabilities, as any other new parent, will face challenges they had not considered during the pregnancy and early years with their child. The difference for parents with learning disabilities is that as soon as they embark on parenthood they are faced with scepticism from most professional services. Their own parents are often fearful of their ability to raise a child, worrying that they, the grandparents, might have to take over child-rearing responsibilities. In addition to this, many health and social work professionals mistakenly fear for the safety of the unborn child (Ward & Tarleton 2007). In short, such pregnancies tend to be considered a huge risk or even a tragedy, rather than the joyful event experienced by the families of non-disabled expectant parents.

There are pockets of excellence in pregnancy services, notably in Scotland where midwives and health visitors use the CHANGE resources. Porter et al. (2012) discuss a project that developed a resource pack of symbolised (accessible) appointment letters, consent forms, scan documentation and information about labour etc. Midwives used these resources with first-time mothers, without any specific training. Results were largely positive, with mothers stating that the pictures helped them to understand some of the difficult concepts involved in pregnancy, such as spina bifida. Midwives were also largely positive about the resources, although they would have welcomed initial training in how to communicate with people with learning disabilities.

Once the child is born, parents report feeling under extreme scrutiny, often feeling that they are being assessed due to an assumption that their child will be neglected. In these cases, parents actively avoid seeking help for minor problems. This has the unfortunate consequence of meaning that they are usually in crisis by the time that they seek help or are reported to services as a cause for concern.

The *Framework for the assessment of children in need and their families* (Department of Health 2000) provides comprehensive guidance for working with families in need; however, social work assessors still find it difficult to work with some parents with learning disabilities. The framework is prescriptive in the time allowed for parenting assessment, yet most parents with learning disabilities need more than the recommended time in order to understand the process and the consequences of some of their responses. Creative methods of communication should be considered to ensure that parents are able to understand what is needed to support their child from infancy to adulthood (Cleaver & Nicholson 2007; Porter et al. 2012).

Good practice guidance was jointly published by the Department for Health and the Department for Education and Skills in 2007. The guidance acknowledged that a multi-agency approach was the key to supporting parents with learning disabilities and their children. The guidance included recommendations for children's and adult services, safeguarding procedures and service commissioners. It acknowledged that communication between schools and parents with learning disabilities is often unnecessarily complex, and urged schools to consider making reasonable adjustments for parents with learning disabilities. These included sending letters out in an audio format and providing stickers that parents could use in homework books rather than providing a signature.

The guidance urges social workers to be respectful of parents, to turn up on time and make enough time available to be able to communicate with parent(s), to be honest and to use simple language. The main messages throughout the guidance are of taking time, being sensitive to communication needs and being proactive, supporting families and avoiding a child becoming 'looked after' by the state.

'Pupil Premium' funding is available to schools to provide extra support to children from disadvantaged backgrounds, including those whose parents have a learning disability. This fund is based on the number of children in a school who receive free school meals. The money is then used to raise the achievement of disadvantaged children. In 2014 this amounted to £1300 per primary school child and £935 per secondary school pupil. Schools can use the money to fund 'virtual school activities' such as providing vouchers for days out during the school holidays and enhancement and nurture groups within school time.

Increasing numbers of people with learning disabilities are choosing to become parents. A timely multi-agency approach is needed to help them and their children achieve their full potential. This approach must be consistent across services. An example of lack of consistency might be the mother who was both praised and criticised for leaving her baby with her mother one day a week while she attended college (Ward & Tarleton 2007, p. 24). Services must be responsive to need, use appropriate communication techniques and choose to believe that families can thrive given adequate support. Where parents with learning disabilities are having difficulties in developing effective parenting skills, they respond best to individual home-based teaching rather than centre-based teaching. Existing parenting packages can be effective with modification. Long-term support may be necessary in order to help families to stay together.

*Implications for practice*

- In January 2016 the government announced its intention to fast-track adoption and fostering processes. Social workers, health visitors and other professionals must be sure that they have supported parents with learning disabilities to be good enough parents before they consider removing their children and freeing them for adoption.

**FURTHER READING**


- McGaw, S. (2000) *What works for parents with learning disabilities* (Barnardos).
- CHANGE, www.changepeople.org/.


## media representation

SEE ALSO **charities and voluntary agencies; discrimination; models of disability**

The media plays a vital part in shaping and informing attitudes towards people with learning disabilities; it includes radio, press, television, books, films, internet and advertising. It has been used to inform, educate, provide entertainment and for political purposes.

The media can be used as a tool to maintain the status quo, reinforcing stereotypical ideas using language and imagery that support certain values, or it can actively challenge these ideas.

The medical model is often the lens through which disability is viewed, with there being a focus on an individual's impairment rather than the person as a whole or a more political analysis of how society and a lack of access and resources disables them (Wood 2012).

Programmes such as Children in Need perpetuate this view with emotive imagery potentially evoking pity and reinforcing a dependence ideology, enabling the 'giving' viewer to feel bountiful and perpetuating a charity-based model as opposed to a rights-based model. Within this context, the term 'carer' has become synonymous with self-sacrifice and martyrdom, implying that the disabled person is a burden and cause of suffering for those around them rather than a more political analysis which would recognise the need for adequately paid support and recognition of the rights of disabled people to live as independently as possible.

More positively, the media has played an important role in exposing the abuse and mistreatment of people with learning disabilities, from the documentary *Silent Minority* programme aired in the International Year of Disabled People (1981), depicting the grim institutional abuse of people with learning disabilities in long-stay hospitals, through to the BBC1 *McIntyre Undercover* and the *Undercover Care – Winterbourne View* programmes, both of which exposed abuse by showing staff violently assaulting and denigrating people with learning disabilities. These types of programmes have effected change by bringing the hidden aspects of the lives of people with learning disabilities to the attention of the general public.

Negative and stereotypical language can still be seen in the media, with terms such as sufferer, courageous, and normal appearing in the national press when writing about disability. This language reinforces discrimination and adds to the imagery which is woven into the consciousness from childhood, often equating disability with evil or badness, such as Captain Hook in *Peter Pan* or Doctor No in James Bond films (Barnes 1992). However, in recent times books more frequently include positive imagery of characters showing how their impairments can enhance as well hinder their ability to get things done. Most notably, *The Curious Incident of the Dog in the Night-time* explores a period in the life of a teenager who has autism, as he sets out on a journey to understand why a dead dog was found in his garden.

There are still very few mainstream films about people with learning disabilities; often people with autism are a focus with the themes of genius and social isolation being juxtaposed together in films such as *Rain Man* (1988), *The Girl with the Dragon Tattoo* (2011) and *A Brilliant Young Mind* (2015).

Over the last ten years there has been greater representation on mainstream TV, with characters with learning disabilities appearing in programmes such as *Eastenders, Call The Midwife, Glee, Mr Tumble* and, more controversially, Channel 4's *The Undateables.*

What we see, hear and read about in the media is decided by a small group of individuals who are influenced by their own values and are generally in privileged positions in society. Ofcom's 2005 report *The representation and portrayal of people with disabilities on analogue and terrestrial television* found that the lack of disabled people employed in the industry had implications for the power of disabled people to influence how they are portrayed in the media; this is amplified for people with learning disabilities who are still further underrepresented.

The Foundation for People with Learning Disabilities has produced guidelines on how they would like people with learning disabilities to be shown. Some issues raised in *We want to be seen and heard* (Foundation for People with Learning Disabilities 2014b) include consideration of what language is used in programmes and to avoid using derogatory terms. It was also considered to be important to depict a variety of people with learning disabilities, not just people with the more identifiable conditions such as Down syndrome. People with learning disabilities wanted their presence on a range of programmes as well as having long-term roles in stories that focus on the complexity in their lives, not simply their disability. The report also highlighted the need for actors with learning disabilities to play the part of characters with learning disabilities.

The internet has opened up far greater access for people with learning disabilities to be involved in producing information and stories about themselves. There are a multitude of information clips on YouTube as well as dramas, arts-based programmes, animations and campaigning information pieces.

*Implications for practice*

- Practitioners need to ensure that people co-produce any media productions in partnership with people with learning disabilities.
- When involved with the media, practitioners need to ensure that programmes give a rounded picture of people and not only focus on their impairments.
- Practitioners need to be aware of perpetuating negative stereotypes through using inappropriate language and images.

**FURTHER READING**

- Shakespeare, T. (1994) Cultural representation of disabled people: dustbins for disavowal? *Disability & Society*, 9(3), 283–299.
- Barnes, C. (1992) *Disabling imagery and the media: An exploration of the principles for media representations of disabled people*, http://disability-studies.leeds.ac.uk/files/library/Barnes-disabling-imagery.pdf.

## menopause

SEE ALSO **healthcare needs; healthcare services**

Ward's (2002) summary of research on the menopause in women with learning disabilities demonstrated an initial focus on when it occurred, identifying that this was at a younger age than for the general population, and even earlier in women with Down syndrome. Later studies were beginning to place far greater emphasis on the impact of the menopause on individuals.

As with other areas, the physical and emotional impacts of the menopause on women with learning disabilities will be similar to the general population. They may experience hot flushes, night sweats, mood changes etc.; however, their individual experience and responses to these 'symptoms' will be impacted by their perception, understanding and ability to communicate this to those supporting them.

Evidence also suggests that the menopause and its symptoms, like other women's health issues (including menstruation), are often not talked about with women with learning disabilities, and behaviours that might indicate the menopause are not distinguished from other causes by carers who recognise the need for better training and education tools to support women at this stage of their lives (Willis, Wishart & Muir 2010).

*Implications for practice*

- It is important to recognise the potential impacts of the menopause on individuals and discuss this with them using appropriate communication strategies in order to help them understand, prepare for and manage the process.
- It is vital to consult and liaise with the person's GP who will provide health advice and help to decide on the most appropriate treatment or support (the GP may need support to relate their approach to a person with a learning disability).

**FURTHER READING**

- McCarthy, M. & Millard, L. (2014) *Supporting women with learning disabilities through the menopause: A resource pack* (Brighton: Pavilion Publishing).

## mental capacity

SEE ALSO **advocacy; mental health; profound and multiple learning disabilities; safeguarding; sexuality**

Mental capacity is the ability to make decisions; this could be decisions concerning everyday life such as when to get up and what to eat, or more serious decisions such as whether to go to the doctors and what medication to take. Mental capacity also refers to our ability to make legal decisions such as agreeing to have medical treatment, get married or write a will.

The Mental Capacity Act (MCA) 2005 provides a framework for considering an individual's ability to make a decision and how, if they lack capacity, to best support them. The MCA has five clear principles and applies to adults over the age of 16 in England and Wales:

- A presumption of capacity: every adult has the right to make his or her own decisions and must be assumed to have capacity to do so unless it is proved otherwise.

- The right for individuals to be supported to make their own decisions: in practice, this means ensuring that people are given all appropriate help to understand the decision in question, taking time and using communication methods that the person understands. Practitioners must be able to demonstrate that they took all reasonable efforts to enhance capacity prior to making a decision as to whether someone has or lacks capacity.
- That individuals must retain the right to make what might be seen as eccentric or unwise decisions.
- Best interests: where a person lacks capacity to make a decision, anything done for or on their behalf must be in their best interests.
- Least restrictive intervention: anything done for or on behalf of people without capacity should be the least restrictive of their basic rights and freedoms.

There may be a number of circumstances where an individual's capacity to make a decision may be questioned:

- The person has a mental disorder (see Mental Health Act 2007).
- The person has made several unwise decisions.
- You believe the person is being coerced into making a decision.
- The person is suggestible and open to manipulation.
- Personal knowledge of an individual where you may recognise someone is struggling to understand a decision.

When working with people with learning disabilities, there are common scenarios that occur in practice where an individual's capacity may be questioned.

- Where to live, and contact and support from family and others.
- Managing money.
- Sexual relationships (see Forced Marriage and Learning Disability Guidelines 2013).
- Engaging in legal agreements such as tenancy agreements.
- Medical treatment.

When considering a person's capacity, it should be decision-specific; a person may lack the capacity about one issue but not about others.

A person can lack the capacity to make a decision at the time it needs to be made and regain it later – the loss of capacity may be partial and/or temporary and it can change over time. Illness and stress may play a role in a person's ability to make a decision at a particular point in time and may not be a factor at a later date. Tools have been developed to help practitioners assess capacity in common scenarios identified above.

Capacity assessment will generally be carried out by the person providing the care or treatment of an individual. This may include a member of staff providing support for someone with an eating disorder who is refusing to eat and a doctor deciding whether a person can make a choice about their treatment.

Capacity requires that a person can:

- Understand and retain the information relating to the decision in question.
- Use that information as part of a process in making the decision.
- Be able to communicate the decision.

**best interest decisions**

If a person has been assessed as lacking capacity, then any action taken, or any decision made for or on behalf of that person must be made in his or her best interests.

The person who has to make the decision is known as the 'decision-maker' and normally will be the carer responsible for the day-to-day care (including care staff, relatives or friends), or a professional such as a doctor, nurse or social worker where decisions about treatment, care arrangements or accommodation have to be made.

While a person has capacity but fears losing it, they can appoint an 'attorney' to make decisions for them if they become incapable of doing so. This Lasting Power of Attorney (LPA) (previously referred to as Enduring Power of Attorney (EPA)) allows decisions to be made in the person's best interests where the LPA has the authority to do so and the person lacks capacity. If a person has a 'deputy' appointed by the Court of Protection, then they must make decisions in the person's best interests where they have the authority to do so and the person lacks capacity.

Decisions about a person's property or their financial matters must be in the person's best interests but can only be made by an attorney appointed under an LPA or EPA, a court-appointed deputy or the Court of Protection itself.

Certain decisions must never be made on behalf of a person who lacks capacity. These are called 'excluded decisions' and include decisions regarding marriage, divorce and civil partnership.

If a person who lacks capacity needs to be kept in a care home or hospital because it is in their best interests, then additional safeguards may apply. These are called the Deprivation of Liberty Safeguards (DoLS), and there is additional guidance about them in a separate Code of Practice (Ministry of Justice 2008a).

**what is 'best interests'?**

The law gives a checklist of key factors which decision-makers must consider when working out what is in the best interests of a person who lacks capacity. This list is not exhaustive, and you should refer to the Code of Practice for more details.

- It is important not to make assumptions about someone's best interests merely on the basis of the person's age or appearance, condition or any aspect of their behaviour.
- The decision-maker must consider all the relevant circumstances relating to the decision in question.
- The decision-maker must consider whether the person is likely to regain capacity (for example, after receiving medical treatment). If so, can the decision or act wait until then?
- The decision-maker must involve the person as fully as possible in the decision that is being made on their behalf.
- If the decision concerns the provision or withdrawal of life-sustaining treatment, the decision-maker must not be motivated by a desire to bring about the person's death.

The decision-maker must in particular consider:

- The person's past and present wishes and feelings (particularly if they have been written down).
- Any beliefs and values (for example, religious, cultural or moral) that would be likely to influence the decision in question.
- Any other relevant factors.

As far as possible the decision-maker must consult other people if it is appropriate to do so and take into account their views as to what would be in the best interests of the person lacking capacity, especially:

- Anyone previously named by the person lacking capacity as someone to be consulted.
- Carers, close relatives, close friends or anyone else interested in the person's welfare.
- Any Attorney appointed under a Lasting Power of Attorney.
- Any Deputy appointed by the Court of Protection to make decisions for the person.

Anyone making the decision under the MCA must take the above steps, among others, and weigh up the above factors in order to determine what is in the person's best interests. For more information, refer to the Code of Practice (Department for Constitutional Affairs 2007).

**mental capacity advocate**

For decisions about serious medical treatment, certain changes of accommodation and care reviews where the person lacks capacity, and where there is no one who fits into any of the above categories to be consulted, the decision-maker must consider whether they need to involve an Independent Mental Capacity Advocate (IMCA). Decision-makers must also consider involving an IMCA in decisions involving adult protection issues, even if there is someone who fits into any of the above categories who could be consulted.

*Implications for practice*

- In a risk averse culture there can be a tacit assumption that it is acceptable to pursue an assessment of capacity in a wide variety of situations, without adequately considering the implications for a person with a learning disability. These may include the psychological impact of feeling out of control of key areas of their lives and subject to the decisions of people who have power over them. Workers need to be clear that an assessment is justified and necessary, and not use assessments arbitrarily or simply to allay their own anxieties.

- It is essential that decisions around capacity are reviewed and that an individual is given the opportunity to challenge outcomes.

**FURTHER READING**


- Department for Constitutional Affairs. (2005) *Mental Capacity Act 2005 Code of Practice* (London: TSO).
- Hardie, E. & Brooks, L. (2009) *Mental Capacity Act 2005: Implications for people with learning disabilities* (Kidderminster: BILD).
- Hardy, S. & Joyce, T. (2013) *The Mental Capacity Act and people with learning disabilities* (Brighton: Pavilion Publishing and Media).
- Brown, H. & Marchant, L. (2013) Using the Mental Capacity Act in complex cases. *Tizard Learning Disability Review, 18*(2), 60–69.


## mental health

SEE ALSO **assessment; behaviour; discrimination; healthcare needs; healthcare services; loss and grief; mental capacity**

Mental health is a vital aspect of our wellbeing and should be considered as something more than just the absence of a 'mental health problem' – as a 'state of wellbeing in which an individual realises his or her own abilities, can cope with the normal stresses of life, can work productively and is able to make a contribution to his or her community' (World Health Organization 2014).

On this basis, everyone has mental health 'needs', and all of us experience changes in our mental health state influenced by social, personal, financial and other factors. A minority of people may experience mental health 'problems' to such a degree that they may be diagnosed as having a mental illness or disorder. It is estimated that at least one in four people will experience some kind of mental health problem each year (Mental Health Foundation 2007). Mental health can therefore be seen as continuum where mental wellness is seen as a positive attribute, but conversely mental ill health is seen as a negative experience.

Mental disorders are traditionally categorised into those which are extreme forms of 'normal' emotions such as anxiety and depression (neurotic), and those in which a person will have an altered sense of reality such as hallucinations or paranoia (psychotic). The most common mental health disorder is anxiety and depression, while more severe mental health disorders such as schizophrenia or bipolar disorder are experienced by much fewer people. All will affect the way that individuals think, feel and behave, and while diagnoses are grouped together, the experience and presentation of the condition will be different for each individual.

Mental wellbeing affects people of all ages, and emotional and psychological distress should not be dismissed in children and young people as it has the potential to profoundly impact on their development as well as their wellbeing, which can cause more profound and enduring problems in their adult lives.

Most people are able to manage their mental health disorders through a range of 'interventions' including medication, therapy, lifestyle and the development of coping mechanisms. For some this will mean a recovery with no subsequent problems, while for others there may be times when they 'relapse' and require more intensive intervention and support, sometimes in a hospital setting.

Some individuals are more likely to experience mental health issues due to a range of both permanent and temporary vulnerabilities. These can include biological factors, personal characteristics, economic status, stressful life events, limited social networks, and physical health and wellbeing.

People with learning disabilities experience mental health in the same way that the general population do; however, they are more likely to have a mental health illness or disorder, with some studies suggesting that as many as 50 per cent of the population with learning disabilities have indicators of a psychiatric condition (Azam, Sinai & Hassiotis 2009). This figure should not be a surprise when considering the World Health Organization statement of wellbeing (above), with people with learning disabilities often having minimal opportunity to attain these skills and functions. Additionally, people with learning disabilities have increased biological (e.g. consequence of genetic condition), psychological (e.g. identification of having a learning disability), social (e.g. stigma and social exclusion) and developmental (e.g. communication) factors that impact on their mental health more than the general population (Cooper & Simpson 2006). People with learning disabilities and a mental health disorder are sometimes referred to as having a dual diagnosis, although this term has other meanings in mental health services (for people with additional substance use issues), so should be used with caution and clarity.

There is a general understanding that mental illness is under-diagnosed in people with learning disabilities, and while the figure quoted here is 50 per cent, there are some variances in prevalence estimates of mental ill health in people with learning disabilities. This can be explained in part by the methods used and the sample groups studied, but may also be due to the difficulties in the assessment and reporting of mental health issues by individuals due to processing and communication difficulties. These difficulties also have a significant impact on people with learning disabilities having their mental health needs first recognised, and then addressed.

Recognition of a mental health issue is an important first step in being able to effectively manage difficulties and seek support. People with learning disabilities may not be able to process and understand feelings of low mood, anxiety or altered perception, or might be unable to communicate this in order to seek support. Carers and staff supporting people with learning disabilities may also not have an understanding of mental health issues, or a positive attitude towards them, and so may not understand the significance or importance of assisting an individual with this area of their life

Similarly, assessment of mental health difficulties in a person with learning disabilities can be a complex process as many of the tools that aid diagnosis rely on the individual to report their feelings and experiences. To assist in appropriate identification, a number of specific assessment tools for mental health in learning disabilities have been developed such as the Psychiatric Assessment Schedule for Adults with Developmental Disabilities (Moss et al. 1998) and the Learning Disabilities version of the Cardinal Needs Schedule (Raghavan et al. 2004).

Consideration of an individual's mental wellbeing is vitally important in more general assessments to counter the possibility of diagnostic overshadowing which is highly evident when identifying mental health issues in people with learning disabilities. This is where signs, symptoms and behaviours etc. are attributed to the individual's learning disability with no recognition of any potential mental health issue.

Care should also be taken when assessing and meeting the needs of people who display behaviour that challenges. There can be a range of functional explanations for such behaviours (e.g. pain, communication, needs not being met), but it is important to consider mental wellbeing as a possible explanation because changes in a person's behaviour are key indicators used to identify and assess mental health issues in people with learning disabilities.

Of course, if mental health needs are not addressed and supported appropriately, then more significant problems could be encountered in the longer term.

Intervention and services for people with learning disabilities will follow similar pathways to that of the general population and may include medication (e.g. antidepressants or antipsychotics), psychological interventions (e.g. cognitive behaviour therapy or psychotherapy) or mental health promotion (looking at lifestyle factors or creating positive environments). These will need to be specifically related to the individual and may involve adaptations to accommodate the person's learning disability.

Initial assessment and management of mental illness will usually be in primary care settings with the GP using and coordinating a range of preventative early interventions. If specialist mental health support is required, then assessment and treatment should be implemented under the Care Programme Approach which is required when an individual has a learning disability and a mental health issue (Rethink Mental Illness 2015). Under this framework, a care coordinator should ensure that support and treatment is implemented and reviewed, with all people involved working together with the individual to promote positive outcomes. For children with learning disabilities, specialist support would usually be provided by the Child and Adolescent Mental Health Service.

Despite *Valuing People* (Department of Health 2001) and subsequent reiterations stating that people with learning disabilities should use mainstream mental health services for their mental healthcare needs, as with more general health services, access to and provision of care can fall short of what would be expected. This is commonly put down to the attitudes and lack of knowledge of staff who are not trained or equipped to support people with learning disabilities, and these can to some extent be changed through education, exposure and support (Rose, Kent & Rose 2011). Better training, facilities and partnership working with learning disability services are vital to developing more inclusive mental health facilities.

As for the general population, there may be times when an individual with a learning disability needs hospital treatment due to the severity of their mental health issue and the risks to themselves or others. In these cases the Mental Health Act 2007 should be followed and implemented, but there will need to be a greater emphasis in relation to the individual's capacity and their understanding of processes and safeguards during their ongoing treatment with reference to the Mental Capacity Act 2005.

Some people with learning disabilities will access mainstream mental health hospitals and wards if they require such intensive support; however, there has been a tendency towards provision of specialist learning disability 'assessment and treatment' services for mental health, autism and challenging behaviour. While this should mean more effective and appropriate support, such units have not been without their problems. *Transforming Care* (Department of Health 2012) – the government's national review following the abuse exposed at Winterbourne View – identifies that these units have supported inappropriate placement of people with learning disabilities and mental health needs in hospital environments, too far away from their families and communities and for longer than is necessary. It sets out a programme of commissioning and development of community services within a National Plan (Houlden 2015) to prevent this, which requires coordination and partnership of mental health and learning disability services to meet the needs of individuals in their localities.

*Implications for practice*

- Promotion of mental wellbeing should be a priority when supporting all people with a learning disability. This should mean more than just ensuring that needs are met and include a focus on empowering choice and control with an understanding and promotion of individual likes and aspirations.
- People should be able to develop meaningful relationships and engage in their communities, with employment opportunities particularly attended to. It is also important for individuals to

develop and have access to coping strategies such as physical activity, time alone or relaxation.

- As mental health status can be hard to assess in people with learning disabilities, it is important that staff understand the indicators of possible changes and are alert to any alterations in a person's mood or behaviour, especially when they do not use words to communicate or have difficulty processing or expressing their thoughts, feelings or emotions.
- Care staff should be particularly observant both at times of known vulnerability for the individual and at more widely accepted times such as bereavement or significant change.
- It may be appropriate to have a baseline indication of a person's mental health status and clear plans that include known and possible triggers, as well as any behavioural or other changes that may mean a person's mental health status is deteriorating.
- At these times, additional emotional support should be offered, with extra steps taken to promote positive mental health through encouragement of coping strategies, providing appropriate outlets and seeking medical support where required.
- Where someone is known to have specific mental health needs requiring support from specialist services, there should be clear guidelines and ways of working identified to ensure effective intervention at appropriate times.

**FURTHER READING**


- MIND, www.mind.org.uk.
- RCN. (2013) *Provision of mental health care for adults who have a learning disability* (London: RCN).


## models of disability

SEE ALSO **history; human rights and the disability rights movement; philosophical approaches**

Disability is often defined in negative terms, as some deficit or lack within an individual. Conceptually it is useful to examine this process by considering models of disability in order to reflect upon the experiences of disabled people and examine our own prejudices, assumptions and worldviews.

There have been several models of disability proposed: the individual; the social; the medical; the charity; the welfare; and the administrative models (Finkelstein 1993). However, the general consensus is that there are two main models of disability: the individual model (which includes medicalisation, often referred to as the medical model) and the social model. The main difference between the models is the way in which disability is framed, the locus of responsibility, and thus the approach taken within the model.

- Individual model of disability: within the individual model, the *impairment* of the individual is considered to be disabling. The person with a disability will be compared to a 'normal' person, and any difference will be construed as problematic. In this model, the impairment is seen as a personal tragedy for the person and/or their family. The individual model includes the medicalisation of disability (Oliver 1990). As such, it is commonly referred to as the medical model and the service response is one of curing, making better and treating with medication.
- Social model of disability: this model does not consider the impairment of the individual to be necessarily disabling. Instead this approach considers the *response* to the individual's impairment to be the disabling feature. This response may be at an individual, community/organisation or societal level. Thus the person is not 'disabled' as such. Rather, the disability is socially constructed through interactions with others/society/attitudes/environments. For example, a building accessible only by stairs might be inaccessible to a person in a wheelchair. Therefore they are disabled by the environment rather than their impairment.

Criticism of the social model of disability has suggested it ignores both the intersectionality of other types of societal disadvantage and oppression such as sexism and racism (Marks 1999). Further criticism has been levelled at the binary nature of these models, that there either is an individual response or a social response (Shakespeare & Watson 2001), a feature which was not originally intended (Oliver 1990). It is suggested there is a need to consider a different approach which acknowledges the difficulties associated with living with impairment (pain, sensory difficulties, fatigue) while also recognising the structural oppression imposed upon disabled people (Marks 1999; Wendell 1989). There has been criticism of the social model as a construct of a Western or Neo-liberal society (Wendell 1989). There is an underlying assumption that disabled people must be included in all aspects of life, including productive work. However, this is not a global phenomenon, and it is important to understand that models of disability are just a way of explaining systems and approaches and do not constitute a reality in themselves. They merely offer a way of thinking about phenomena.

Often the most disabling response is structural, at a societal level and attitudinal rather than environmental. While considering disability as an identity is useful as a political tool, to identify with others who share experiences, and when campaigning and raising political awareness, for people with learning disabilities this is problematic. However, people with learning disabilities have often been excluded from the political disability movement and not all people with learning disabilities consider their identity to be one of 'disabled', but of being 'people first'.

The model of disability is important as it will offer a lens through which the individual will be viewed, determine how disability is framed and thus shape the response from services. It is important for practitioners to be aware of the model of disability from which they make decisions. It is also important to consider that this worldview may not be shared by the individual, their family/carer or other professionals. Thus if parties are considering the issue from a different perspective, this may cause friction and disagreement within agreed plans.

*Implications for practice*

- When the medical model is the dominant framework, then the service response will be one of treatment, surgical intervention, curing the individual and easing suffering. If an individual has cerebral palsy, the medical approach may be conductive education, operations to lengthen bones or physiotherapy to develop muscle tone, whereas the social approach may be to offer an electric adjustable wheelchair.
- Often there is confusion between medical *approaches/treatments* and the medical *model*. The impairment of the person may well require a medical response, for example if an individual has

epilepsy, they may require medication and treatment, they may also require consideration of safety with regards to seizure management, yet the response may be framed within a social model perspective. Thus the individual may choose to wear padded hat, wear an SOS safety bracelet and have an identified safety plan. They may choose not to have part of their brain cauterised in an attempt to stop the seizures.

## FURTHER READING

- Swain, J. & French, S. (2008) *Disability on equal terms* (London: Sage).

# p

## parents of people with learning disabilities

SEE ALSO **ethnicity; loss and grief; international perspectives; profound and multiple learning disabilities; transition**

> *I think no other group of people in the world wishes their child to die before they do – but for parents of someone with high support needs it is very worrying that they will be left with no one to make sure they are happy, loved and cherished as full human beings.*
>
> (Towers 2013, p. 7)

Becoming a parent can be a time of great excitement, although many parents also experience feelings of apprehension and anxiety as the birth approaches. The reality of becoming responsible for a small, helpless person, completely dependent on others to meet their every need, can take some adjusting to. While most parents expect such dependency to diminish as the child grows older, parents of babies with learning disabilities may feel initially that they will be solely responsible for their child until they die – as illustrated in the passage from Towers, above.

Antenatal checks might indicate that a baby is likely to be born with a learning disability; however, in some instances the disability will only become apparent at birth or later in life if a child fails to achieve maturational milestones. The attitude of the practitioners who inform the parent of their child's disability has an important bearing on how the parents manage the news. Where pregnancy results in a healthy, non-disabled baby, parents are congratulated on the birth. Where a child is born with a learning disability, parents are all too often greeted with commiseration and sorrow. For example we can think about the difference it would make to a new parent to hear these two phrases, 'Congratulations you have a healthy baby girl' and 'I am sorry to have to tell you that your baby has Down syndrome'. The first example is full of hope and happiness, and the importance of gender is often stated at this time. However, where a child has a learning disability, the message is delivered with less hope and gender is often overlooked as the process of turning the baby into a genderless, eternal child begins.

It is important that professionals inform parents of any disability in a calm and positive way, stressing the things that the child could be capable of as well as informing parents about the support that they might be entitled to. Practitioners who express sorrow or embarrassment when breaking what they consider to be the 'bad' news can have a lasting detrimental effect on the way in which parents perceive their babies.

Parents who are told that their baby has a disability describe feeling a mixture of happiness that the baby is alive, shock and disbelief about the diagnosis, and grief for the loss of the non-disabled child that they expected. This process can be likened to a bereavement and often follows a recognised pattern, from 'why me?' to seeking a cure and even bargaining with God for a miracle recovery. The process of adjustment differs with each parent and may begin all over again at key periods in the child's life, such as starting and leaving school, first love, seeking employment and leaving home.

Adjusting to the news that a baby has a disability can be challenging, as can breaking the news to other family members. Some family members may find it difficult to accept the news. Where family relationships are already strained, grandparents may seek to blame their son-in-law or daughter-in-law for the disability.

Practitioners should be aware of cultural beliefs, because the birth of a disabled child is considered to be a punishment from God or vengeful ancestors in some south Asian and African cultures (Tafirei, Makaye & Mapetere 2013; Hervie 2013). In such instances, care needs to be taken to understand how cultural beliefs might impact on the parents' willingness or ability to accept advice and support.

Parents of children with mild to moderate learning disabilities may find that there is little difference between bringing up their child and bringing up a child without a disability. School days, holidays and transition to college and work all progress as smoothly, or not, as with any other family. However, parents whose children have profound and multiple learning disabilities (PMLD) describe their lives as a battleground between themselves and services, rather than having a normal experience of family life. Care needs to be taken to support families in a person-centred way. Social workers and community nurses must challenge generic policies such as those that restrict the provision of disposable continence pads to three per person per day – evidence shows that the average toilet use is six to eight times a day.

Parents of adolescents and adults with learning disabilities are often misunderstood by professionals who accuse them of being overprotective or reluctant to let their adult child 'move on'. The reality for parents is that for much of the time the family is left to manage alone, with many marriages ending due to pressures of caring for a child with a disability.

In a survey of over 300 parents carried out for the Foundation of Learning Disabilities, the majority had considerable anxieties regarding the future of the children. Many, particularly older parents, have memories of long-stay hospitals and large residential homes and fear that their children will be neglected or worse if they enter 'the care system'. Between 52 and 66 per cent feared that after their death their children would not have their support needs met in a place where they were happy, or with people that they liked, or that decisions would be made in their best interests (Towers 2013).

It is estimated that the number of people with learning disabilities aged over 65 will double in the next 20 years or so. This increasing longevity of people with learning disabilities is a good news story – people are living longer, holding down jobs, becoming parents and living fulfilling lives. However, approximately 60 per cent of people with learning disabilities continue to live with their families, with a third living with family carers being aged 70 or older (Mencap 2002).

Objectives set in *Valuing People* (Department of Health 2001) and developed in *Putting people first* (Department of Health 2007) have begun to change parental opinion, with many younger parents having a better understanding of the developments in learning disability services. The introduction of Direct Payments and Individual

Budgets has led to an increase in numbers of young people with learning disabilities leaving the family home between the ages of 18 and 25. Many parents consider 18 to be the age at which young people leave home for university and expect services to enable a young person with a learning disability to do the same. While it used to be the case that the young person would have to wait until the local authority had a vacancy in a supported tenancy, if they could not live independently, Individual Budgets now offer greater flexibility, enabling them to look at a range of alternative accommodations. This is leading to an anomaly where increasing numbers of siblings with learning disabilities are leaving the family home at a younger age than their non-disabled siblings, many of whom are unable to find work after leaving school or university and are remaining in the family home until their late 20s and 30s.

*Implications for practice*

- Parents of people with learning disabilities need to be given accurate information and support.
- Most local authorities support parents' groups that can offer advice and support to parents. These not only provide opportunities for families to meet and share experiences but can provide a forum for action, for example holding local services to account where they are slow to adapt to changing demographic need.
- A national charity for families with disabled children, Contact a Family, also provides information, support and advice for families.

**FURTHER READING**


- Contact a Family, www.cafamily.org.uk/.
- Towers, C. (2013) *Thinking ahead: Improving support for people with learning disabilities and their families to plan for the future* (Foundation of People with Learning Disability).


## person-centred approaches

SEE ALSO **assessment; care planning; empowerment; personalisation; philosophical approaches**

Services for people with disabilities have historically focussed on meeting identified and eligible 'need', and subsequently developed interventions that aim to reduce the impact of impairment and thus increase independence and participation in communities. Person-centred approaches start from the other end and ask first how people with disabilities want to live their lives, before looking at how this might happen.

Person-centred approaches are rooted in the belief that people with disabilities are entitled to the same rights, opportunities and choices as other members of the community and are concerned with the whole of someone's life, not just their need for services (Sanderson et al. 1997). They challenge the traditional notion of 'independence' by seeing it in terms of choice and control rather than physical capacity to carry out particular tasks. Person-centred approaches go beyond 'needs', as they consider people's aspirations, are not limited by entitlement to services and are not necessarily dependent upon professional involvement.

While the term 'person-centred approaches' is relatively new, it relates to a set of values and ways of working that have roots within much wider historical movements that have challenged the way that people with disabilities are included in society. These include the social model of disability, the inclusion movement and social role valorisation, which all seek to positively include people with disabilities by providing frameworks for rights and independence.

The term 'person-centred planning' has often been used as a way of describing a collection of tools or strategies that can be used with individuals. However, while tools and templates may help to prompt ways of supporting people in a more person-centred way, unless they are used within a person-centred way of thinking and working, they will not have the desired impact. They must be used with the intention of giving people who have learning disabilities more positive control over their lives and making sure that services do a better job of listening to what people who use them really want, and then making sure it happens. 'Person centred planning is a process for continual listening and learning, focussing on what is important to someone now and in the future, and acting upon this in alliance with their family and friends' (Department of Health 2001).

Tools range from those which focus on specific decisions or interventions such as 'working/not working', 'sorting important to and important for' and '4 plus 1 questions' (Helen Sanderson Associates

2016b), to much more detailed processes across a range of aspects of an individual's life and planning for their future such as 'PATH' (Planning Alternative Tomorrows with Hope),or 'MAP' (Making Action Plans) (O'Brien, Pearpoint & Kahn 2010).

Fundamental to person-centred thinking is a change in the way that people with learning disabilities are viewed and a change in the relationship between them and people who are paid to support them. This is helped by a focus on what people like and admire about individuals, and on their aspirations, rather than simply on their needs, and forms the basis of self-directed support and personalisation – which is how health and social care funding and support should be assessed and provided.

There should be an emphasis on people with learning disabilities (and their families) being partners (Duffy & Smith 2007) in the assessment, planning and provision of support at every level and stage of the process. On a care management level, which includes both supporting people to get the help they need and the allocation of resources (Duffy & Sanderson 2005), this includes assessors helping individuals to think about and identify their own dreams and goals, listening to them and acting to help them attain them. On a more direct support level it includes individuals having choice and control over who is employed to support them, with an emphasis on 'matching' the skills and interests of the person being employed with what is important to the person they will be supporting (Helen Sanderson Associates 2016c).

Some people with learning disabilities choose to ask a small group of their friends, families and other significant people to work together with them to help stay in control of their lives, plan to achieve their dreams and help them overcome any barriers (Burke & Ball 2015). These are commonly known as 'circles of support', which are increasingly being used to support person-centred outcomes in communities and employment. Circles of support have also developed as a way of helping people to use their personal budgets to help shape their support and achieve their goals and aspirations (Neill & Sanderson 2012).

Person-centred thinking is not exclusive to working with people with learning disabilities, yet there is a strong tradition of developing these approaches within learning disability services. More recent practice has seen person-centred thinking, and some of the specific tools such as one-page profiles, used and promoted across all services, institutions and communities.

Person-centred thinking, and the tools that are associated with it, are increasingly being used as a way of underpinning the way that services operate internally, with a focus on the development of the relationships between individuals, teams and services (Sanderson & Lepkowsky 2014). This works from the simple notion that having a shared sense of vision and purpose with each member of the team knowing their role, playing to individual strengths and knowing how to work with and support each other effectively ultimately leads to better performance and productivity on both an individual and a team level. Examples might include: 'person-centred supervision' which creates a sense of value and investment in the individual by the organisation; 'positive and productive meetings' which encourage participation and engagement; and developing a team or service PATH which helps to endorse a collective vision and shared purpose of the organisation (Sanderson & Lepkowsky 2014). Person-centred ways of working will be most effective if they are applied across all aspects of service commissioning, design and delivery.

*Implications for practice*

- Working in a person-centred way should shift the balance of power from services to the individual being supported, giving them increased independence through having choice and control and opportunities.
- A person-centred approach should be concerned with what is important to the individual being supported and what support they need to attain this.
- Person-centred ways of working should support and enhance the individual's place in their community, promoting them as a full and active citizen.
- Person-centred plans are only part of a person-centred approach and should be constantly reviewed, developed and maintained.
- Person-centred ways of working should be used to enhance teams and services and develop a culture of person-centred thinking.

**FURTHER READING**

- Cambridge, P. & Carnaby, S. (Eds.). (2005) *Person centred planning and care management with people with learning disabilities* (London: Jessica Kingsley Publishers).
- Community circles, http://community-circles.co.uk.
- Helen Sanderson Associates, www.helensandersonassociates.co.uk.
- Paradigm, www.paradigm-uk.org.
- Sanderson, H. & Lepkowsky, M.B. (2014) *Person-centred teams: A practical guide to delivering personalisation through effective team-work* (London: Jessica Kingsley Publishers).
- Thompson, J., Kilbane, J. & Sanderson, H. (Eds.). (2007) *Person centred practice for professionals* (Maidenhead and Berkshire: Open University Press).

## personalisation

SEE ALSO **adult social care; assessment; history; philosophical approaches**

Personalisation as a concept has been around for two or three decades, but it wasn't until the millennium that it started to gain real momentum both as an ideological approach and a possible policy framework. The four principles of *Valuing People* (Department of Health 2001) – independence, choice, rights and inclusion – summarise the underlying ethos behind the concept of personalisation. These principles, in turn, were drawn from a wealth of work and belief from the 1970s onwards that individuals with support needs should be valued, enabled and have opportunities to participate in ordinary community life and exercise autonomy.

Following the introduction of the NHS and Community Care Act 1990, an emphasis was placed on support in the community as opposed to within large segregated hospitals and institutions, as had previously been the case. In 1990, people were commonly talking about care *in* the community, but care *by* the community was a concept that was discussed less. The separation of care commissioning and care provision that the NHS and Community Care Act 1990 brought with it meant that a culture of professionals developed who were 'in charge of the purse strings' and had the remit to assess, plan and implement or commission care and support that was readily available and could be block-purchased. Although people were being supported, they often lacked choice and control over the services that they received.

*Valuing People* (Department of Health 2001) recommended that children and adults with learning disabilities were to be provided with greater support and opportunity to become more independent and to become more included in their local communities. Following on from this, a registered charity, In Control, was formed in 2003 by a small group of people who were committed to improving the lives of disabled people and their families. They 'pioneered the concept of self-directed support and developed personal budgets as a way for people to take charge of their support...This model (was piloted) across six areas in England – bringing real, sustainable benefits for people with no increase in costs' (In Control 2014). Subsequent government papers further strengthened the agenda that was fast being referred to as the 'personalisation agenda'. *Putting People First* (Department of Health 2007) set out information to support the transformation of social care, as outlined in the health White Paper *Our Health, Our Care, Our Say* (Department of Health 2006). It describes the vision for development of a personalised approach to the delivery of adult social care.

The notion that people could be given the opportunity to direct and lead their own support and oversee their own budgets was a radical move away from one where the state controlled such aspects of a person's life. These ideas of more personalised and individualised support are inextricably linked to those of citizenship. Duffy proposes six keys to citizenship (2010), defining citizenship as being respected, being equal and being different:

1. **Freedom** – the authority to control our own life – being able to make decisions, make mistakes, and make our own way.
2. **Direction** – having a life of meaning, and a plan to achieve that life.
3. **Money** – to live and control our own life.
4. **Home** – a place we can call our home, not just a shelter, but a place where we can have privacy, be with those we love, and where we belong.
5. **Help** – support to do the things we might need help to achieve.

6. **Community Life** – the opportunity to be actively engaged and able to contribute to community life.

In proposing these six keys for citizenship, Duffy offered practical strategies for ensuring that citizenship could include all people, including disabled, very severely disabled and learning disabled people. These keys sit side by side with person-centred thinking, as they ask the same questions and seek the same outcomes.

*Personal health budgets* were introduced in 2014 by the NHS as a way of giving individuals the opportunity to manage their own care in a way that suits them – they consist of an amount of money which can be used to support an individual's identified health and wellbeing needs. This is in addition to *personal budgets*, which are intended to support an individual's social care needs. These are mechanisms that allow the principles of self-directed support and personalisation to become a reality for people who have support needs. However, it is imperative to remember that 'Personalisation is fundamentally about better lives, not services. It means working with people, carers and families to deliver better outcomes for all. It is not simply about changing systems and processes or individualising funding through personal budgets and direct payments, but includes all the changes needed to ensure people have greater independence and enhanced wellbeing within stronger, more resilient communities' (TLAP 2016).

*Implications for practice:*

- Those who support people with learning disabilities need to understand the importance of citizenship, belonging and autonomy, and that the personalisation agenda has positive implications for social justice.
- The range of funding options for achieving a life which is self-directed is broad and at times complicated in terms of administration and legality. People with learning disabilities and their families and carers may need support to navigate the system.

**FURTHER READING**

- Department of Health. (2010) *Personalisation through person-centred planning* (London: DH).

- National partnership transforming health and care through personalisation and community-based support, www.thinklocalactpersonal.org.uk/.

## philosophical approaches

SEE ALSO **human rights and disability rights movement; terminology; history; discrimination; ethnicity**

The 1960s saw the beginnings of a radical change in how services for people with learning disability were structured, particularly in the UK, Canada, the USA, Scandinavia, Australia and New Zealand. Reports into the treatment of people in long-stay mental health hospitals revealed that at best the lives of people with learning disabilities were being wasted, and at worst they were being abused by the people who were paid to care for them.

The status of isolated, congregated and segregated services was challenged by a series of abuse scandals and some high profile research experiments such as that undertaken by Jack Tizard. The Brooklands experiment (1958–1960) involved moving children from the Maudsley hospital into eight-bedded 'family group homes', cared for by 'houseparents'. The staff were required to provide care and developmental opportunities, usually through play, to the children, as opposed to the mainly custodial and regimented approach provided in the large hospital setting. The progress of the children was compared to that of a control group who stayed in the hospital. The experiment revealed that small-group living and opportunities to develop meaningful relationships with a small group of care givers enabled the children to progress much more quickly than those in the control group. The experiment is credited as being highly influential in the development of community and day services for people with learning disabilities.

Although people with learning disabilities had only been subjected to forced group living for less than a century the seeds of fear and prejudice had been sown deeply into the consciousness of most Western societies. Communities became fearful of having people with learning disabilities present in their midst and the move from hospital back to community living has proven to be very slow.

**normalisation**

A set of principles for community living referred to as 'Normalisation' began to emerge in the 1960s. Bengt Nirje (1969) defined the principle as 'making available to the mentally retarded patterns and conditions of everyday life which are as close as possible to the norms and patterns of the mainstream of society' (p. 19). He went on to outline his eight principles of Normalisation, which are briefly outlined here:

1. A normal rhythm of the day, for example getting up and dressed rather than languishing in bed no matter how profoundly disabled a person might be.
2. The normal routines of life, as other people have them, for example going out to work or for leisure, not having all your needs met in the same place.
3. A normal rhythm of the year, holidays and days of personal significance.
4. Normal developmental experiences of the life cycle, for example children should experience warmth and nurturing and be guided by a small number of adults. Nirje was adamant that infants, teenagers and adults with 'mental retardation' should not be 'confined to the same institutions'. Stating that 'young people's socialization and impressions of life should be gained as much as possible through contacts with normal rather than deviant society' (p. 20).
5. Choices, wishes and desires should be considered. People should not be forced into large heterogeneous groupings that make communication difficult. He cited research from groups of 18 to 30 year olds who described the need for services and outings to be offered to small homogeneous groups to enable similarly minded people to enjoy things together.
6. The opportunity to live and move in mixed-sex groups and experience sexual relationships in a manner that is 'commensurate with normal restraints', going on to state that 'the mildly retarded sometimes suffer loneliness that has no sense... they may be better off married' (p. 21).
7. Normal economic standards, including child allowance, old age allowances or minimum wages for work undertaken in sheltered workshops.

8. Physical facilities, for example schools, hospitals and group homes, should be of a size that is commensurate with the locality in which they are based and should be similar in size to those used by ordinary citizens.

Critics of Normalisation suggested that the philosophy was flawed; some suggested that it was a white Eurocentric idea, which required all people to conform to the norms of Western societies. Others criticised the concept because it failed to realise that people with learning disabilities could never be 'made normal', which suggests a lack of understanding of the principles. Oliver (1999) suggested that Normalisation compounded the disabling effects of society by encouraging people to conform to normative appearance and behaviour, although there is no evidence to support this in Nirje's work.

**social role valorisation**

Academics continued to develop empirical research showing the benefits of supporting people with learning disabilities in ordinary settings. Wolfensberger (1972) is credited for developing Normalisation into the social science theory that became known as Social Role Valorisation (SRV). He argued that people should be afforded the 'good things in life'. Critics such as Brown and Smith (1989) asked, 'Who defines the good things in life?' However, Wolfensberger was clear from the outset that the 'good things' are:

- Absence of imminent threats of extreme privation.
- To be viewed as a human being and treated with respect.
- To be treated justly and have a say in the important issues affecting one's life and good health.

**wounds and death making**

Wolfensberger believed that services 'wounded' people with learning disabilities rather than improving their lives. For example antipsychotic and other psychotropic medication is prescribed to many people who do not have a diagnosis of psychosis simply to subdue a person and manage behaviour that we find challenging (Sheehan et al. 2015). Such prescribing appears to alleviate 'symptoms', that is, reducing the behaviour by subduing the individual, although most experts now agree that such behaviour is symptomatic of a deeper problem existing between the person and their relationship with their environment. The mis-prescribing of anti-psychotic medication does nothing to help us understand what the behaviour was trying to tell us. Most such medication has side effects that necessitate other drugs to offset these effects. These combinations can have damaging long-term physiological effects. Wolfensberger went on to say that in some instances the overuse of medication may actually hasten death, a process that he termed 'Death Making'.

**model coherence**

In addition to considering how individuals are supported, Wolfensberger also developed a method for analysing how human services are structured, paying particular attention to the support of people with disabilities and other devalued groups. The programme analysis of service systems (PASS and PASSING) tools enable a detailed analysis of how and where services are situated and staffed, and how these might impact not only on the people who use the service but also upon members of communities who might make assumptions about the service and the people who used it. These analytic tools enable service providers to compare provision to the ways in which ordinary people live their lives. This notion of model coherence highlights just how far removed most services are from the ordinary patterns of living that Nirje recommended. PASSING assessments, which must be undertaken by trained providers, assess any type of human service provision, from homes for older people to hostels for ex-offenders. The key to model coherence is to examine how closely the lives of service users mirror the lives of other people of a similar age, ethnicity, social status etc. who inhabit a similar location.

**ordinary life principles**

At this time, John O'Brien and Connie Lyle (1987) developed an arguably more user friendly treatise on the development of human services. The '5 Service Accomplishments', sometimes referred to as 'Ordinary Life Principles', state that people must have:

- Community presence – living and participating in activities with members of the community.
- Choice – the right to make real choices, big and small, about things that happen in their lives.

- Competence – learning to achieve things for themselves, big and small, from dressing to learning a skill for a job, with assistance where necessary.
- Respect – to be valued as a full citizen, having respect for themselves as well as from others.
- Community Participation – a wide variety of friendships, including with non-disabled people.

O'Brien's influence cannot be overstated; his work proved pivotal in the development of person-centred planning in the UK and the USA. He argues passionately for the *inclusion* of people with learning disabilities throughout societies, rather than their continued hidden existence in separate, specialist services. The effect of this approach can be seen in the closure of large long-stay institutions, inclusive education and the development of *Valuing People* (Department of Health 2001), *Valuing People Now* (Department of Health 2009a) and *Valuing Employment Now* (Department of Health 2009b). His person-centred planning tools 'Planning Alternative Tomorrows with Hope' (PATH) and 'Making action plans'(MAPS) (O'Brien, Pearpoint & Kahn 2010) are widely used in learning disability services in the UK and the USA.

*Implications for practice*
- People with learning disabilities can achieve many of the lifestyle choices taken for granted by their non-disabled friends and neighbours.
- People may not need to seek support from services, but when they do these services must be sure to respond in a way that enhances the person's life rather than diminishes it.
- Ordinary life principles and SRV are now widely used across human services, including mental health services.

**FURTHER READING**

- Race, D.G. (2006) *Social role valorisation and the English experience* (London: Whiting & Birch).
- The SRV Journal, www.srvip.org/journal_general.php.
- O'Brien, J., Pearpoint, J. & Kahn, L. (2010) *The PATH & MAPS handbook: Person-centred ways to build a community* (Toronto: Inclusion Press).

## physical disabilities

SEE ALSO **healthcare needs; healthcare services; profound and multiple learning disabilities**

People with learning disabilities can have additional physical impairments that may or may not be a result of their specific condition. These can be congenital or acquired following illness or injury, as would be the case for anybody else. A person with a learning disability may need additional support to adapt to any acquired disability. Specific physical impairments commonly related to learning disabilities are cerebral palsy, profound and multiple learning disabilities, and dysphagia (Mansell 2010).

Cerebral palsy is caused by damage to the area of the brain that controls the muscles, and can result in muscle stiffness or weakness, uncontrolled body movements and balance and coordination difficulties. Difficulties can occur in one or more parts of the body, with each affected in a different way. Physiotherapy can help people with some of the physical difficulties they may experience; where communication is affected, a speech and language therapist may be appropriate – each person should be assessed as to best intervention for them. The severity of the condition will vary from person to person, as too will its impact both physically, with pain a significant feature, and emotionally, with depression not uncommon. It should be noted that cerebral palsy is not a learning disability but can be accompanied by a learning disability.

People with profound and multiple learning disabilities will usually have high support needs in many areas, including mobility, due to the nature of their physical impairment. Moulded wheelchairs are identified in the ***profound and multiple learning disabilities*** entry as a positive intervention to assist with physical needs, but other considerations are also required.

We all need to move and change body position in order to maintain and improve positive health, including having a good posture. Where people are unable to move or reposition themselves over a sustained period, there is a greater risk of body distortion, which is sometimes seen as an inevitable consequence of profound learning and physical disabilities. This is in fact not the case, and postural care uses 'the right equipment and positioning techniques to help protect and restore body shape' (Mencap no date).

Postural care should form an important part of the care and support that people with profound disabilities receive from their immediate carers following training by an appropriate qualified professional. 'Raising our sights' (Mansell 2010) recognised this importance, with failure to address individual needs in this area resulting in significant health complications and extreme pain.

Dysphagia is a condition that affects a person's ability to swallow, with difficulties possible in the mouth, throat or oesophagus (NHS Choices 2016a). This can lead to complications such as dehydration, malnutrition and aspiration, each of which have potentially serious consequences.

While evidence is limited, it is thought that there is a higher proportion of people with learning disabilities that experience swallowing difficulties than the general population, and this is more common in people with profound physical impairment and with cerebral palsy as well as their learning disability (Harding & Wright 2010).

Dysphagia might be considered if an individual takes a long time to eat their meals, they cough or choke a lot on food or drink, report a feeling of something being stuck in their throat, regurgitate or if there are any other unusual signs or symptoms when eating. Investigation is usually under the direction of a speech and language therapist who will also make recommendations to improve eating and drinking that may include changing eating behaviours, thickening fluids, changing posture and positions when eating, and training and supporting carers.

*Implications for practice*

- Individuals with physical needs should be supported holistically to maintain and improve health with support from therapists as required.
- People supporting individuals with learning disabilities should be alert to possible physical issues, including dysphagia.
- Families and carers may need training in order to provide safe care to individuals with physical needs, for example in postural care or supporting someone to eat and drink.

**FURTHER READING**

- Cerebral palsy.org.uk, www.cerebralpalsy.org.uk/.
- Postural care information, www.mencap.org.uk/posturalcare.

## professional practice

SEE ALSO **healthcare needs; healthcare services; interprofessional practice; person-centred approaches**

Professional practice refers to people who are paid to support people with learning disabilities, and includes those who require a qualification in order to undertake their specific role and those who have no such requirement. In order to understand the development of professional practice, it is necessary to have knowledge about the context of care and how this has developed over the last 30 to 40 years.

People with learning disabilities have always lived at home and in communities, but, historically, significant numbers were also placed into institutional care, often in large long-stay hospitals away from their families and communities. The NHS & Community Care Act 1990 thankfully prompted a move away from this form of care, with 'residents' gradually moved out, usually into small group living houses dispersed across towns and cities with a view to integrated community living. These properties were typically managed by local authority and NHS services, but with an increasing drive away from such provision support is now more commonly provided by a range of private companies and charitable/not-for-profit organisations. These can be very small, local organisations, or national and multinational companies. More recent moves to support individuals to live an independent life in their own homes through personalisation and personal budgets mean that support is also available through direct employment by the person with a learning disability, or 'bought-in' care through a dedicated care agency.

Changes in care delivery for people with learning disabilities brought an acknowledgement that staff providing support to them required better training and qualifications, including the skills to work in partnership with users and carers in a multidisciplinary way (Department of Health 2001). This was identified as particularly important for unqualified staff that made up the biggest proportion of the workforce, not just to increase standards of care and support but to afford greater status and recognition to the vital work they did. A succession of training and qualification frameworks (NVQ/LDAF/QCF) have subsequently been implemented, these provide opportunities for professional development and support progression into more senior roles and higher level awards.

Many people who work in these roles, or who have family experiences, decide to develop a career supporting people with learning disabilities at a more advanced level in jobs that require specific professional training and qualifications. Routes to achieve these qualifications are usually based within the higher education sector, requiring minimum standards of entry qualifications and leading to professional registration. Registration exists in order for professions such as nursing to set and maintain standards of education, training, conduct and performance (Nursing and Midwifery Council 2016) in order to protect the public, maintain the standing and reputation of the profession and ensure high-quality care.

While there are some specialist learning disability qualifications, many have generic training, with individuals then choosing their field of practice on qualification and developing specialist practice through experience and further training.

The nursing profession in the UK is divided into four 'fields of practice': adult; mental health; children and young people; and learning disabilities. All nurses would be expected to have a level of knowledge and understanding about how to support people with learning disabilities, as they will undoubtedly work with them in the course of their practice; however, learning disability nurses focus on the needs of this population.

Whereas other fields are specific to age (adult/child), learning disability nurses work with people from 'cradle to grave' and so might work in a range of settings from schools, nurseries and children's hospitals, to community adult teams, mental health wards and care homes. As such, they need to be equipped with a diverse range of knowledge and skills, and while other fields might emphasise intervention to improve health at a time of need, a learning disability nurse's focus is on 'improving or maintaining a person's physical and mental health; reducing barriers to them living an independent life; and supporting the person in living a fulfilling life' (Healthcare Careers 2016). Training is across a three-year programme of undergraduate or postgraduate (sometimes shorter) study which contains both theoretical and practical elements.

The social work profession is focussed on supporting individuals, families and communities to improve outcomes in their lives through an emphasis on empowering them, and advocating for social justice and change. It is a general qualification, meaning that practitioners can work with people across all ages and communities, including people with learning disabilities. Work can be statutory (social workers act as agents of the state usually within legal frameworks of social welfare, safeguarding etc.) or in a range of other settings such as residential, advocacy or early intervention etc. (Prospects 2016).

Training for social workers is currently based in higher education, with both undergraduate (three years) and postgraduate (two years) courses which include practice placements in social work settings. Recent changes to social work training have encouraged those with a high-level first degree to enter the profession through shortened programmes such as Frontline (2015) and 'Step up to social work' (Department for Education 2016) which are focussed on those wishing to work with children and families.

There are examples of courses that have combined the professional elements of both learning disability nursing and social work into a single integrated qualification. These courses recognise that the rights and needs of people with a learning disability are not clearly divisible into health or social care, and believe that effective support can be best achieved through a more holistic approach. They emphasise the shared knowledge, skills, values and practices of the two professions, and assert that understanding and integrating the differences gives practitioners the best basis for professional practice in partnership with people with learning disabilities, their families, support staff and the multidisciplinary team. Courses are usually three years at undergraduate level, leading to professional qualification as both a learning disability nurse and social worker, with practitioners working in any of the settings that might be expected of the single professional groups.

Teaching is another profession regularly associated with people with learning disabilities, particularly in relation to special educational needs. While many individuals with learning disabilities are supported in mainstream education, there are still a number of 'special schools' where teachers will only support those with learning disabilities. Training for teachers is generic, with individuals who wish to work in special schools usually developing their experience within the mainstream context before looking to work specifically in special education and undertaking further training and qualifications (National Careers Service 2016).

There are a range of other professionals who might regularly be involved in supporting individuals with learning disabilities in generic or mainstream services. These might include physiotherapists, speech and language therapists, occupational therapists, doctors, dentists etc. It is important that these professionals have a good awareness and understanding of the impact a learning disability may have on an individual, particularly in relation to additional or specific health needs, communication, promoting understanding and compliance etc. As with teaching, these professions may also provide opportunities for specialist practice with people with learning disabilities, but these require qualification in the general practice of the profession prior to specialising over a period of experience with and/or additional study of the specific needs of people with learning disabilities.

The way in which many of these professions provide specialist support has changed alongside the way residential services have developed. Institutional care and segregated services meant that many of the professional services were provided in segregated environments, and while this is still the case in some smaller units (which usually support individuals in a secure environment), the move to community provision has promoted access of people with learning disabilities to generic services.

Specialist provision is therefore intended to be focussed on those with the most significant needs offering targeted support, often in multiprofessional community teams, to assess and plan required care, provide therapeutic intervention and ensure immediate carers have the knowledge and skills to implement required support. Further still, specialist learning disability practitioners may help improve access to generic services by supporting not only the individual but also the staff in order to make adjustments to their practice to effectively meet the needs of the diverse population.

Alongside the change in roles and services offered, there has been a significant shift in the approaches taken to the support of people with learning disabilities as a shared value base has emerged within all professions based on principles of empowerment, equality and choice. This has had a significant impact on professional training and education, with challenges to the way people with disabilities are viewed in society leading to more person-centred approaches to working (O'Brien & O'Brien 2002) and an emphasis on 'doing with' and 'enabling to', rather than 'doing for'.

*Implications for practice*

- There is a range of residential and support services, and specialist professional groups who work with people with learning disabilities; services and staff should work together, acknowledging and utilising the different skills and approaches they have, in order to provide the best support to individuals.
- Staff working with people with learning disabilities should be supported to access the required training and development to improve their knowledge and experience and provide high-quality support.
- There are a range of options and professional qualifications that people can take if they want to develop a career supporting people with learning disabilities.
- All professional practice should focus on working in partnership, with people supported to improve their outcomes.

**FURTHER READING**


- Gates, B., Fearns, D. & Welch, J. (Eds.). (2015) *Learning disability nursing at a glance* (Oxford: Wiley Blackwell).
- National Career Service, http://nationalcareersservice.direct.gov.uk/Pages/Home.aspx.
- Williams, P. (2009) *Social work with people with learning difficulties* (Exeter: Learning Matters).


## profound and multiple learning disabilities

SEE ALSO **assistive technology; communication; healthcare needs; mental capacity; physical disability; sensory disability; syndromes**

The acronym PMLD has variously been used to describe both people with Mild Learning Disabilities and people with Profound and Multiple Learning Disabilities, which can create significant difficulty in understanding and requires clarity in relation to terminology used. It is the latter group of people that are identified here, along with recognition that this term is increasingly being replaced by Profound Intellectual and Multiple Disabilities (PIMD). People in this group have a profound learning disability alongside other physical or sensory disabilities (or both) that might result in severe limitation in self-care, continence, communication and mobility (World Health Organization 1997).

While people with profound and multiple learning disabilities have always formed a significant proportion of the total population of people with learning disabilities, evidence shows there is an increasing number. This can be explained in part by rising birth rates and people with learning disabilities living longer (as with the general population), but there are also more premature babies surviving, and advances in medical procedures and technologies that mean that children who might otherwise not have survived are living to adult life (Emerson 2009). The percentage of people who are dependent on medical technologies and have complex healthcare needs is also increasing (Carpenter 2000).

There are many myths and misconceptions surrounding people with profound and multiple learning disabilities. These include being given prognoses of very limited life expectancy and an inability to interact with other people and their surroundings. While it is true that people with profound and multiple learning disabilities do have a higher mortality rate than the rest of the population (Mansell 2010) and often have significant difficulties in communication, there is also evidence to show that with the correct levels of support, people with profound and multiple learning disabilities survive and thrive into adulthood. Research also shows that they can enjoy friendships and engage in meaningful activities (Prime Minister's Strategy Unit 2005).

Many people with profound and multiple learning disabilities have additional health needs that can be a part of their disability, such as respiratory problems resulting from congenital lung abnormalities, or that can result from some of the difficulties that their disability presents, such as repeated respiratory infections due to limited mobility and poor nutritional health. They are also more likely to have epilepsy, dysphagia (swallowing difficulties), gastrointestinal conditions or musculoskeletal issues. Some people with profound and multiple learning disabilities may have additional conditions such as autism, Rett syndrome or Down syndrome.

Some people with profound and multiple learning disabilities will demonstrate signs of *tactile defensiveness* (TD) (an inability to tolerate touch); this can be extremely distressing for the individual and their carers because of the large amount of personal care that they will receive. It is possible to assist people with TD by observing which types of touch can be tolerated and gradually building an intervention to increase tolerance (Bradley 2012). It is also important to observe whether an individual demonstrates signs of TD with all of the people who provide care and support for them or whether this relates to a specific person.

Support for people with profound and multiple learning disabilities has greatly improved across a range of areas in recent years:

- Bespoke moulded wheelchairs and body braces not only significantly improve an individual's health, they also provide social benefits because people in a seated position can be perceived to be more able than a person lying prone, which was the case for many people in the past.
- Intelligent wheelchairs are becoming available for people with profound and multiple learning disabilities; these enable individuals to move around their homes and schools more easily.
- Smart communication aids which enable specific decision-making are more readily available.
- Medical interventions have improved, such as those that ensure adequate nutrition (for example percutaneous endoscopic gastrostomy, or PEG) and keep people healthier and help prevent illness.

There is evidence that some of these developments are more accessible and available to children with profound and multiple learning disabilities than adults, with suggestions that public attitudes that value the protection of children consequently mean there is lower investment in technologies that could give some independence to adults with profound and multiple learning disabilities, for example in making simple choices or moving to different locations in a building (Mansell 2010).

The introduction of personal budgets has enabled many children and adults with profound and multiple learning disabilities to enjoy a better quality of life. Families access these budgets in different ways. Some enjoy the freedom of controlling budgets, developing personalised support and recruiting personal assistants (PAs), while others seek support from provider agencies to help them to manage the challenges of becoming an employer.

Supporting a person with profound and multiple learning disabilities is a skilled occupation. PAs may be required to assist with tasks as varied as providing oxygen therapy and tube-feeding to supporting a person to use assistive technologies to aid communication. Although it is understood that families are often the experts in the needs and best ways to support individuals with profound and multiple learning disabilities, it should not be left to them alone to train the next generation of support workers. There is still insufficient commitment by central government and local authorities for the provision of effective training programmes to enable PAs to gain necessary skills (Mansell 2010).

Support for families of individuals with profound and multiple learning disabilities is vital, and as young people with such complex needs reach adulthood there is a substantial shift in the support that may be offered to families. Medical care and treatment that would have been overseen and managed by a single paediatrician supported by dedicated and familiar staff both in the hospital and community may be replaced by a number of specialities, and necessitate not just the introduction of one, but many, medical support services, depending on the individual's needs. Daytime activity in colleges, day centres, outreach or employment may not replicate the regularity and consistency of school, with families having to adapt their routines around changes in caring requirements. Short break (respite) provision might not match the levels of support provided by children's services, or might be provided in a different way, with carers coming into the home rather than the young person being supported in a specialist unit.

In common with other groups of people who rely on others for personal support, individuals with profound and multiple learning disabilities are at a higher than average risk of physical and sexual abuse (Brownridge 2006; Powers et al. 2008).

Observation of everyday routines can be key not only to keeping people free from abuse but to helping them to be able to communicate with friends and family. By paying careful attention to small gestures or repeated behaviours, family, friends and PAs can begin to understand individual needs, wants and preferences. It is possible to help people to develop and use signs to demonstrate need. For example if 'Sara' has no verbal communication but screams repeatedly and stops screaming when she receives a drink, it might be concluded that she is using her scream to ask for a drink. She may bite her hand to signify hunger. By supporting her to learn some simple signs, maybe a small movement in her head or a sign that she makes onto someone else's hand, she could begin to develop a 'vocabulary' rather than relying on behaviours that might be used to label her as challenging.

Developing an understanding of the individual's communication is also vital to ensure that all support takes place in accordance with the Mental Capacity Act 2005. No matter how profound a disability is suspected, capacity should be presumed and people supported to understand information using all means possible in order to help them make decisions. Where necessary, family and independent advocates should be used to support decision-making processes within a best-interest framework.

*Implications for practice*

- Individuals with profound and multiple learning disabilities and their families may require additional support to negotiate their way through care services, particularly as they transfer from child to adult services.
- Commissioners and service providers will need to develop ways of working that are flexible to respond to the needs of individuals with highly complex care requirements, by increasing the skills of the care workforce to meet individual needs in a person-centred way.
- Assistive technologies should be explored that offer greater communication and independence to individuals with profound and multiple learning disabilities.

**FURTHER READING**

- PMLD network, www.pmldnetwork.org/.
- Lacey, P. & Oyvry, C. (Eds.). (2012) *People with profound & multiple disabilities: A collaborative approach to meeting complex needs* (Oxon: Routledge).

## puberty

SEE ALSO **safeguarding**

In general puberty will commence between the ages of 9 and 15 and take place over a number of years, but for people with learning disabilities, the process of puberty may commence later and take longer. The physical and hormonal processes, combined with emotional responses, can be a challenging and difficult time for young people with learning disabilities, and they may need additional support to understand what is happening to them. Puberty will usually bring an awareness of one's own sexuality, which can be an added confusion and frustration for young people with learning disabilities who may have limited opportunities for self-exploration.

Where many children will learn and explore their bodily changes and sexuality in discussion with their peers, for a variety of reasons, including communication difficulties and lack of opportunity to meet outside of school, this is not always possible for children with learning disabilities – meaning further restrictions and a very 'formal' version of explanations from sex education at school or from parents.

Children with disabilities are at an increased vulnerability to abuse (Murray & Osbourne 2009), and this can increase as they experience puberty and begin to develop and express their sexuality. Knowledge and understanding of social rules and appropriateness of public and private behaviours may be limited, and this might make them more vulnerable to exploitation from others.

There can be some reticence by care staff to address the needs of children and young people in relation to puberty and sexuality, and it is important to identify that the law protects workers when providing legitimate sex education within an approved care plan (Home Office 2004).

*Implications for practice*

- Supporting a child with learning disabilities through puberty and exploring their sexuality will not be any different to a child without learning disabilities in terms of the information that needs to be given; however, this must be presented in a way that is accessible to aid their understanding and might include using pictures or models (The Children's Learning Disability Nursing Team, Leeds 2009). It might also mean creating opportunities for them to meet and discuss changes with their peers, with the increased opportunity this provides for them to develop relationships and learn from their own experiences.
- In order to protect children and young people from abuse, it is vital to empower them with information and practical skills to recognise and manage abusive situations or relationships. This may include developing role plays to help prepare them and protect themselves by knowing how to react and then report concerns.

**FURTHER READING**


- The Children's Learning Disability Nursing Team, Leeds. (2009) *Puberty and sexuality for children and young people with a learning disability: A supporting document for national curriculum objectives* (Leeds: NHS Leeds).

# r

## radicalisation

SEE ALSO **criminal justice & forensic services; serious case reviews**

Nicky Reilly, a young man with Asperger syndrome, was the first convicted would-be suicide bomber in the UK to have a learning disability. Reilly was radicalised through his use of the Internet. Although much of his contact with terrorists was made via a PC in his bedroom, he was also known to connect and speak with terrorists in Jordan and other Islamic countries while attending a learning disability day centre.

Reilly had a history of mental health problems in addition to Asperger syndrome and developed an obsession with tall buildings and warfare following the bombing of the World Trade Centre in New York in September 2001. Having disclosed to a therapist his wish to join Hamas, he attempted to bomb the Giraffe restaurant in Exeter in 2008. Internet records show that Reilly was influenced by a man calling himself Adal Khan, although this is believed to be a pseudonym. It is clear that Khan and others groomed Reilly by befriending of an otherwise isolated young man. The term 'mate crime' is sometimes used to describe this befriending a person in order to lead them into crime or to perpetrate a crime against them (Grundy 2011).

The *Prevent strategy* (HM Government 2011) and *Channel duty guidance* (HM Government 2015a) seek to help parents, schools and other services to recognise signs or indicators of potential radicalisation. These include change in dress or appearance, desire to change a Christian or given name, changes in socialisation, having new friends or withdrawing from previous friendships. The strategies aim to re-educate individuals prior to them becoming detached from their communities of origin.

*Implications for practice*

- People with autism and/or learning disabilities tend to have fewer friends than their non-disabled peers. It is therefore essential to support them in understanding friendships.
- Parents and carers should be mindful of friendship patterns as well as changes in patterns of behaviour.

**FURTHER READING**

- HM Government. (2011) *Prevent strategy* (London: Crown Copyright).

## research

SEE ALSO **charities and voluntary agencies; empowerment; history**

People with learning disabilities have been the subject and object of much research in the last century or so, as various groups have sought to understand the physical and societal causes of their disabilities. Early research problematised people with learning disabilities and concentrated on what could be done about, with, or to them, so that they might contribute to society rather than being a perceived threat to it. For example while medical research published in the *British Medical Journal* (BMJ) explored issues such as hereditary conditions and the best ways to treat or cure what was then called feeblemindedness, it also reported on the therapeutic impact of work upon feebleminded people. One such paper, produced by the National Society for the Employment of Epileptics, discusses the relative merits of outdoor work, finding that light outdoor work is slightly more beneficial for women than for men (BMJ 1904). Much of the research produced in the early 20th century was not undertaken by physicians but by social scientists, who were extremely influential on policymakers. During this time, social hygienists such as Alfred Tredgold and Mary Dendy, alongside Frances Galton, a cousin of Charles Darwin, became very influential. Much of their research employed poorly interpreted Darwinist theories together with emerging gene theory to propagate the myth that if left unchecked (i.e. allowed to live and bear children), people with learning disabilities would ultimately cause the downfall of British society.

Happily, history has moved on from this approach, and by the middle of the last century people with learning disabilities began to be supported to publish their own accounts of their lives. One of the first to be published described the life of Joey Deacon, a man with cerebral palsy who after spending a happy childhood with his family was admitted to hospital care following the deaths of his main family carers (Deacon 1974). As case history research, Deacon's story provides a wealth of evidence about the everyday lives of people with disabilities growing up in post-war England. The mere fact that the work was written was a major achievement because Deacon's speech was so severely affected by his condition that only his friend Ernie could understand him. Ernie couldn't write so had to interpret Deacon's words to another friend to type. The book was followed by television documentaries and an appearance on the children's television programme *Blue Peter*.

Other case studies followed, and the histories and voices of people with learning disabilities slowly began to emerge in the tumult of research produced by non-disabled people (Atkinson 2004). However, a question remained about the control of the research agenda, with much of the published research being produced by academics. Even today, people with learning disabilities are more likely to be invited to participate in the research of others as advisors and collaborators, rather than as leaders and controllers of research projects (Bigby et al. 2014).

This is because government departments, large organisations and interest groups are largely responsible for setting the agenda and providing the funding of most learning disability research. Organisations such as the Joseph Rowntree Foundation, the National Institute for Health Research and others now require that any group wishing to bid for learning disability research grants must include people with learning disabilities as research partners. This requirement has enabled organisations such as Mencap, the Foundation for People with Learning disabilities, CHANGE and others to begin to steer the agenda from within. While it is obviously beneficial that individuals and groups of people with learning disabilities are now included in research in a variety of ways, their status and degree of involvement within research partnerships is not always clear in final reports.

Walmsley (2001) used the term 'Inclusive research' to encompass a range of terms such as 'participatory', 'emancipatory' and 'action research' as applied to research that includes people with learning disabilities as active contributors rather than respondents. A study describing the co-production of the development of accessible information for women with learning disabilities who have been raped is an example of collaborative action research (Olsen & Carter 2016). This is an example of a woman with a learning disability, Catherine Carter, building on expertise that she had gained as a focus group participant. Using this and previous research experience, she co-led and co-authored a study of her own choosing.

It is difficult to gauge how much small-scale research is currently being undertaken by people with learning disabilities, as co-authorship of studies remains problematic. Many studies report the inclusion of people with learning disabilities, yet contributors' names are often omitted from published reports. Some academic authors state that this is to protect the identities of research participants and their families, particularly if the research is of a sensitive nature such as rape and domestic violence. However, this remains a questionable and potentially paternalistic stance, as participants with learning disabilities could adopt a research nom de plume, as some non-disabled authors have done in the past.

While lack of ownership of the products of one's own research might be problematic for most researchers with mild to moderate learning disabilities, there is another group who remain largely excluded from the research agenda. People with profound and multiple learning disabilities (PMLD) are still rarely included as research partners. Mencap has recently concluded a three-year consultation exercise aimed at overcoming some of the barriers faced by people with profound and multiple learning disabilities who might want to be involved in decision-making processes. The resulting 'Involve Me' resources are a valuable tool for ensuring that people with profound and multiple learning disabilities are meaningfully involved in research and decision-making activities.

*Implications for practice*

- There is little doubt that collaborative research between people with learning disabilities and others is important.

- Care must be taken to consider how such research is undertaken; this should include challenging academic paradigms of data collection, analysis and reporting.
- Research findings must be made accessible for people with learning disabilities.

**FURTHER READING**

- Jackson, M. (2000) *The borderland of imbecility: Medicine, society and the fabrication of the feeble mind in late Victorian and Edwardian England* (Manchester: Manchester University Press).
- Mencap, 'Involve Me' resources, www.mencap.org.uk/involveMe.

## restrictive practices

SEE ALSO **behaviour; behavioural approaches**

Much of the emphasis in recent behavioural approaches, and central to the concept of positive behaviour support, is a reduction in the use of restrictive practices used in order to manage behaviour that challenges. However, there is recognition that there may be occasions when such an approach is required in order to protect the health and safety of the person presenting with the behaviour and/or those around them.

Any restrictive practice used should be done with consideration to a range of 'tests'. It should be: the last resort – in that all other interventions should have been exhausted prior to use; least restrictive – where there are a range of possible interventions; reasonable and proportionate – to the danger or threat posed by the behaviour; for the minimum possible duration – with ongoing assessment aimed at ending the intervention; and in the best interests of the person supported, gaining consent in the form of an advanced directive where it is possible to do so (Department of Health 2014b). The There Is No Alternative (TINA) principle is often used to determine the appropriateness of any restrictive intervention.

All such intervention should take place within a clear care plan, agreed by the multidisciplinary team and governed by the legal framework incorporating the Mental Capacity Act 2005, Mental Health Act 2007 and the Deprivation of Liberty Safeguards 2009.

When talking about restrictive interventions at the point of behavioural crisis, these usually fall within three categories.

Physical intervention is any form of taking hold of a person in order to control or manage their behaviour. This includes where the intervention is done by people, or mechanically using equipment such as emergency response belts. Any physical intervention should be done by appropriately trained staff, with a number of 'models' now having been developed that place such action in a positive behavioural support (PBS) framework and which use techniques that are designed specifically for people with learning disabilities that cause no pain and minimal discomfort to the individual (British Institute of Learning Disabilities 2014).

Using the environment to restrict individuals at a time of crisis is called seclusion; this is a term mired in confusion when in fact the legal standpoint is quite clear. Seclusion should not form part of any therapeutic behavioural intervention and can only be used as an emergency response in a clinical setting (where appropriate facilities, support and monitoring protocols can be adhered to as required under the Mental Health Act 2007 and the accompanying code of practice) (Department of Health 2015a). In fact, any withdrawal of interaction or isolation of an individual outside of these occurrences are constituted as a punitive action and are therefore unlawful. Seclusion does not simply relate to the locking of people in a confined area, and, significantly, if the person believes they cannot leave the area, or that they cannot access interaction, then this will constitute an illegal act of seclusion. In a community setting, seclusion cannot take place and environmental controls should only be considered in a one-off emergency to maintain safety, with future, more appropriate responses assessed and implemented as part of a care plan. The term 'time out' is often used (and confused or conflated) with seclusion, and again forms part of a punitive approach to behaviour modification and should be avoided.

Medication can be used as a chemical restraint that 'tranquilises' the individual, making the behaviour less intense. Use in this way, at times of crisis, should be seen only as a short-term intervention to reduce immediate risks and not as part of ongoing treatment (Department of Health 2014). The medication used is usually a benzodiazepine and is often described as 'PRN' or 'as required', and is given at the time of the behaviour to prevent deterioration and/or reduce intensity. Use in community settings should be written into a care plan with clear guidelines as to when and how they should be given. Confusion does exist between the use of medication in this way, and as a way to control symptoms (i.e. subdue the behaviour) on a longer-term basis.

While the use of any of these approaches in the appropriate context and within clearly defined parameters is a valid way of supporting people with learning disabilities, and offers protection for support staff from legal redress, misuse should be considered abuse and dealt with very seriously.

A wider consideration of restrictive practice is now encouraged and supported by legal precedent, *P v Cheshire West and Chester Council* and *P and Q v Surrey County Council* (2014), in that any intervention that restricts an individual's movement, action or freedoms (not just at times of behavioural crisis) when compared to the general population should be considered as a breach of their basic human rights. Lord Justice Hale's helpful commentary on a Supreme Court ruling that 'a gilded cage is still a cage' (Penny & Exworthy 2015) emphasises that however well-meaning or necessary an intervention, it is still a restriction and so individuals should be offered legal protection in order to promote their rights and to be free from any form of abuse. This is not designed to prevent supporting agencies from offering appropriate restrictions (such as locking the door to prevent a person with a learning disability leaving the house if they do not have an understanding of road safety, or may be vulnerable to crime) but to ensure that these are done with a clear rationale, supported by evidence and legally determined using the principles identified through this entry.

Closer attention has been paid to the support of people with learning disabilities (and/or autism) who display behaviour that challenges (and/or have mental health issues) in restrictive environments since the Winterbourne View scandal was exposed as part of the BBC's *Panorama* series (*Undercover Care* 2011). Subsequent reports that investigated the wider context of this abuse (Department of Health 2012; Bubb 2014) reaffirmed the findings of the Mansell report (2007) in finding that this particular cohort of people were being grouped together in 'specialist assessment and treatment units', often many miles from their homes and families, and were living there indefinitely. The reports identify that not only is it more likely for institutional abuse, such as that at Winterbourne View, to occur in these units, but that the majority of individuals placed in them are done so because there are not appropriate services in their local authority communities, and not because they actually need such restrictive support. The government has set out a 'National Plan' to develop models of appropriate community support in order to reduce the need for such specialist 'in-patient' provision and therefore close over half the current number of 'beds' by 2019 (Houlden 2015).

In order to achieve this, the plan states that there needs to be 'a shift in power to individuals and a change in services ... to see people with a learning disability and/or autism as citizens with rights, who should expect to lead active lives in the community and live in their own homes just as other citizens expect to' (p. 5).

*Implications for practice*

- People with learning disabilities should be supported in least restrictive environments with an emphasis on providing support that minimises the chances that the need for restrictions will arise.
- Any restrictions imposed on an individual's natural environment, human rights, or liberties should be clearly identified and documented with a clear statement of the reasons why such restrictions are necessary and supported by evidence of legal and best interests decisions.
- Any additional restrictive practice deemed necessary as a result of a person's behaviour should be documented within a care plan with clear direction as to when and how this should be implemented. This should be reviewed on an ongoing basis.
- Any restrictive action taken should be in the individual's best interests and with regard to principles of last resort, least restrictive reasonable and proportionate intervention.
- All discussions in relation to the restriction of an individual should include them and/or their family and advocates seeking consent for proposed interventions.

**FURTHER READING**

- British Institute of Learning Disabilities (BILD), www.bild.org.uk (factsheets on chemical restraint; key considerations in physical interventions; the use of seclusion, isolation and timeout).
- Department of Health. (2014) *Positive and proactive care: Reducing the need for restrictive interventions* (London: DH).

## risk

SEE ALSO **advocacy; assessment; mental capacity; safeguarding**

Risk and hazard are terms used interchangeably, but it is important to know the difference. A hazard is 'anything which may cause harm to an individual' (HSE, 2015); whereas risk is 'the chance (high or low) of someone being harmed by the hazard, and how serious the harm may be', (Health and Safety Executive 2015). Harm is defined in the Children Act 1989 as 'ill-treatment or the impairment of health or development', but there is no distinction made in the legislation between 'harm' and 'significant harm'.

Assessing risk usually involves a matrix and scoring system (actuarial risk) which considers the likelihood of the incident occurring and the likely impact of the event. For example, if the weather forecast is for rain, it may be very likely that an individual will get wet if they go out in the rain, but this will have little real impact, they can get dry and there will be no long lasting effects. If the forecast, however, is for sunshine, the person may burn, they may suffer heatstroke or they may eventually be more at risk of skin cancer. We can reduce risk by encouraging the individual to wear appropriate clothing and using sun protection where necessary.

Some risks are considered to be worth taking for the benefit. If the person is going to play football, then although it may rain and the person will get wet, they cannot play football in a waterproof jacket, trousers and wellies! So we manage the risk, and at certain times we take risks. When weighing up the risks we consider the positive aspects – sunshine improves our mood, it helps us produce vitamin D – against the negative ones. Exercise keeps us fit, and team exercise can help us to make friendships and avoid social isolation. In assessment terms, playing football when rain is forecast could be considered to be positive risk-taking because the potential benefits outweigh the potential risk.

However, the consequences of the risk may be too high to allow the individual to take the risk. An individual who is allergic to tree nuts needs to be protected against ingesting them in any form, as the likely outcome might be death – therefore the risk would be more serious and we cannot let this happen even one time.

Some risks need a professional assessment, for example the risk of choking needs to be risk assessed by an individual competent in dysphagia, usually a speech and language therapist but other practitioners may be competent. The most important issue is that the individual is 'competent' to risk assess. Practitioners must not act outside their 'scope' of practice but seek advice and refer on to someone else if they feel unable to assess.

Some risk must be managed urgently, for example if an individual is displaying behaviour which is labelled as challenging and they are posing a risk to themselves or others then this must be managed immediately before other longer-term interventions are put in place. In this case, such 'reactive strategies' may be put in place but the intention will be for a short-term plan while other assessments and plans are developed. Risk assessments must therefore be reviewed regularly; they should have a review date on them, and this may be on an hourly, daily, weekly, monthly or longer basis.

Risk is an important concept within health and social care. It is impossible to eliminate totally but needs to be managed effectively so that people with intellectual disabilities experience the 'good things' in life. We can take one of two approaches to risk and risk management: we can either be risk averse – so advocating protection and safety; or we can take a positive approach to risk management – whereby we balance risk with danger and allow individuals to make mistakes, make what we may consider to be 'bad' decisions and hopefully learn from their mistakes.

Risk is considered at different times as part of any assessment. Before a home visit, we may be assessing risk to the individual, but also to ourselves as practitioners – are there any dangerous dogs, or does the individual or a family member have a history of violence or aggression towards professionals? What is the environment like? Is it safe to visit alone after dark? Is it safe to leave your car on the street? Managing these personal safety risks is essential. Check with the organisation – what safety strategies are in place? Do they have a buddy system, a lone working policy, an alarm system? The risk should be documented, thus for future visits all professionals can be prepared. However, if this is a first visit or the person has not been seen for a while or their circumstances have changed, then the risk must be reassessed.

In terms of clinical risk, for example when administering medication we are risk assessing in terms of the individual's mental health, the safety of the environment, the infection control, the risk of adverse reactions or side effects, but we also have a duty to maintain vigilance with regard to other safety concerns that we may have. It is important to make every contact count in terms of child sexual exploitation, domestic abuse, hate crime and hate incidents, issues with neighbours, physical health, mental health and wellbeing, isolation and other vulnerabilities. Getting risk assessment wrong can have fatal consequences; therefore, assessments must be completed thoroughly and with support from other professionals and key stakeholders such as family, friends or circles of support.

Families are often sources of risk, and relationships should be monitored discreetly. Safeguarding procedures need to be at the forefront of your mind, as the information you are getting may lead you to be suspicious about risk – if you have any concerns, then raise them with your line manager and make sure this is documented. If an individual discloses abuse, then be aware that evidence must be preserved and also of the emotional impact on the individual.

*Implications for practice*

- Risk assessment has been in the spotlight recently in response to child sexual exploitation (CSE) cases and serious case reviews. The Chief Social Workers for both Adults and Children and Families have stressed the need for vigilance and diligence in risk assessment but also have highlighted the importance of risk assessment being based on clinical and professional judgement, involving 'experts' and supervisors, discussion of cases and accurate record-keeping.
- The Care Act 2014 encourages positive risk-taking rather than adopting an overprotective attitude towards people with learning disabilities. In such instances, practitioners should search for

protective factors, such as personal resilience and family or community support, and also consider hazards that might threaten individual wellbeing.

## FURTHER READING

- Health and Safety Executive, www.hse.gov.uk/risk/faq.htm.
- Letter from the Chief Social Worker for Children and Families to Local Authority Directors of Children's Services, Chief executives and Lead Members, www.gov.uk/government/publications/tackling-child-sexual-exploitation-letter-from-isabelle-trowler

# S

## safeguarding

SEE ALSO **empowerment; hate crime; mental capacity; risk; serious case reviews; sexuality**

### adults

Safeguarding is about protecting vulnerable adults and children from abuse or neglect. The term vulnerability has been widely used in the context of safeguarding. The core definition of 'vulnerable adult' came from the 1997 consultation 'Who Decides?', issued by the Lord Chancellor's Department, and is a person who 'is or may be in need of community care services by reason of disability, age or illness; and is or may be unable to take care of him or herself, or unable to protect him or herself against significant harm or exploitation'. This definition of an adult covers all people over 18 years of age. *No Secrets* (Department of Health & the Home Office 2000, p. 9) was the first guidance on developing and implementing multi-agency policies and procedures to protect vulnerable adults from abuse, it was reviewed in 2009 with the key issues identified as the need for greater empowerment and participation of vulnerable adults in the safeguarding process. *No Secrets* has now been superseded by the Care Act 2014.

The Safeguarding Vulnerable Groups Act 2006 identifies that people are vulnerable whenever they are in circumstances whereby another person can exercise power over them in the form of legitimate authority. This legislation covers the barring of unsuitable people from working with children and vulnerable adults.

Practitioners need to consider the use of the term 'vulnerable adult'; it is argued that the term promotes the idea that society's primary responsibility should be to act as custodians and protectors, not to respect and promote the freedoms of people with learning disabilities, and that it also displaces accountability by locating the vulnerability within the person, not their life situation and circumstances (Long, Roche & Stringer 2010).

There is an inherent tension between the ideas of 'rights, empowerment and choice' and that of 'safeguarding and protection'; there needs to be a balance between preventing abuse and minimising risk without taking control away from individuals, and responding proportionately if abuse or neglect has occurred.

Children and adults with learning disabilities may be at increased risk of abuse for a number of reasons; these include:

> Communication issues: people may have limited communication skills and be unable to tell someone what is happening to them, or their communication is interpreted as 'challenging behaviour' rather than a sign that they might be being abused.
>
> Dependency: people with learning disabilities may be dependent on a wide range and number of people, which increases the risk of abuse.
>
> Fear and lack of power: people with learning disabilities are often taught to comply with the wishes of other people, especially those who have power over them. They may lack in confidence and self-esteem to be able to challenge abuse and poor practice.
>
> Education and understanding: people with learning disabilities may not have received sex education or support in understanding finances as well as a lack of awareness of their rights.
>
> Capacity: some people with learning disabilities may lack the capacity to give informed consent to particular activities such as sexual intercourse and therefore do not understand what is being done to them and cannot construe it as abuse or rape. (Brown & Craft 1989)

In order to address these issues, practitioners need to actively engage people with learning disabilities in work around sex education, rights-based work, self-advocacy, building self-esteem and ability to resist compliance.

The key pieces of legislation supporting safeguarding are the Care Act 2014, Equality Act 2010, Safeguarding Vulnerable Groups

Act 2006, Mental Capacity Act 2005, Sexual Offences Act 2003, Public Interest Disclosure Act 1998, Human Rights Act 1998 and Mental Health Act 2007. No single piece of legislation gives specific protection against abuse in law; various acts may give power in different situations and unlawful acts may be dealt with through criminal law.

There have been a number of high-profile cases of abuse and people with learning disabilities resulting in serious case reviews; some are related to institutional abuse such as Winterbourne View where secret filming by BBC's *Panorama* (*Undercover Care* 2011) revealed the psychological and physical abuse and torture of people with learning disabilities in an assessment and treatment hospital. The abuse went unchallenged over a protracted period of time despite numerous complaints about the treatment of the people that lived there. It was unnoticed by the Care Quality Commission who inspected the organisation shortly before the television programme was aired. However, a serious case review was undertaken following the programme, resulting in the hospital and three other services run by the same company being closed down. Hate crime also links to safeguarding, and serious case reviews have been carried out in relation to this concerning both adults and children.

Abuse of people with learning disabilities can also frequently be perpetrated by family members and carers within their own homes. It is only relatively recently that there has been a more systematic collection of data by the Health and Social Care Information Centre whereby it is possible to identify and analyse in greater depth how abuse impacts on people with learning disabilities.

All local authorities are required to have adult safeguarding policy and procedures which practitioners must be familiar with. The Care Act 2014 has clearly laid out the responsibilities of local authorities in respect of safeguarding. These are:

- A statutory duty to set up Safeguarding Adults Boards, which should include the local authority, NHS and police, and whose role it is to oversee adult safeguarding within the local authority.
- A duty to make enquiries when there are suspicions that an adult is experiencing abuse.
- To make safeguarding enquiries a corporate duty for councils.

- To make serious case reviews mandatory when certain triggering situations have occurred and the parties believe that safeguarding failures have had a part to play.

**children**

Children with learning disabilities, like adults, have a heightened vulnerability to abuse, for the reasons outlined previously. Safeguarding is a term which is broader than 'child protection' and relates to the action taken to promote the welfare of children and protect them from harm. Safeguarding is everyone's responsibility. Safeguarding is defined in *Working together to safeguard children* (HM Government 2015b) as:

- Protecting children from maltreatment.
- Preventing impairment of children's health and development.
- Ensuring that children grow up in circumstances consistent with the provision of safe and effective care.
- Taking action to enable all children to have the best outcomes.

The main legislation that covers child protection is the same for all children; practitioners need to be familiar with the Children Act 1989 and 2004, *Working together to safeguard children* 2010 with amendments 2013, 2015 (HM Government 2015b). The government has also produced specific guidance relating to the safeguarding of children with disabilities highlighting the need for good communication with children and young people, provision of adequate support to families and the need for sex education and training for staff working with disabled children (Murray & Osborne 2009).

*Implications for practice*

- As a practitioner you have a moral obligation, a right and a duty to raise with an employer any instance of malpractice, negligence or unprofessional behaviour and any matter of concern relating to delivery of services or care which are detrimental to children's, service users' or carers' interests.
- Child and adult safeguarding is a complex area of work; practitioners need to ensure that they are aware of local policy and procedures and are sufficiently trained to work in this area.

- The ethical challenges are to balance the rights of people with learning disabilities to take risks and have control over their own lives while ensuring justice and protection from harm.

**FURTHER READING**

- Brown, H. & Craft, A. (1989) *Thinking the unthinkable: Papers on sexual abuse and people with learning difficulties* (Family Planning Association Education Unit).
- Hughes, L. & Owen, H. (2009) *Good practice in safeguarding children: Working effectively in child protection* (London: Jessica Kingsley Publishers).
- Mantell, A. & Scragg, T. (2008) *Safeguarding adults in social work* (Learning Matters).

## sensory impairments

SEE ALSO **autism; communication; healthcare needs; profound and multiple learning disabilities**

People with learning disabilities are as many as ten times (visual) and eight times (hearing) more likely to have impairments affecting these senses than the general population, with one in three thought to have some sort of sensory deficit.

Sight is a vital sense that affects a person's ability to learn, communicate and interact with people and their environment (Pilling 2011). The same is true of hearing, which enables similar interactions with the environment and other people to enhance communication (Brennan 2013). Having poor or restricted sight or hearing therefore reduces an individual's independence, increases isolation, restricts communication and interaction, and can potentially have a significant impact on their quality of life.

Significant sight loss is thought to affect one in ten people with learning disabilities (Royal National Institute for the Blind 2016). For those with more severe disabilities or where sight loss may be a feature of their condition (e.g. Down syndrome), this may be unavoidable, but for others it may be preventable or at least possible to slow progression if conditions that cause such irreversible damage (e.g. glaucoma) are identified and treated earlier.

Recognition and identification of sight issues is perhaps the major issue when considering visual impairment in people with learning disabilities. As with other health conditions, people with learning disabilities may not be able to recognise or communicate that they are experiencing difficulties with their sight, and if they have always had deficits they may not know that they have a problem. Carers may make assumptions about an individual's need for good sight, if they are unable to read, for instance, or not consider sight issues if there is no presenting reason to do so. They may miss behavioural signs that there is a problem with vision, instead putting it down to other factors or behavioural problems (diagnostic overshadowing).

In addition to those people who have some sight loss, it is estimated that six in ten people with learning disabilities may need glasses (Seeability no date), yet many do not get their eyes checked regularly, for similar reasons to those identified above. This can be compounded by the inaccessibility of the standard eye test to those who cannot read. Assumptions are often made about whether people with learning disabilities will 'tolerate' glasses, yet they should be supported to try them and using a slow introduction may have opportunity for improved vision (Gates, Fearns & Welch 2015).

Improving eye health for people with learning disabilities requires better awareness and education of good eye health and potential sight issues with both individuals and the people that support them. This should include information presented in a way that can be understood and with opportunity to fully explore and understand it. Accessing an ophthalmic test at the intervals recommended for all children and adults will also mean regular checks are made and assessment done of the possible benefits of an individual wearing glasses, as well as a referral to more specialist eye and vision specialists if appropriate. As with other professions, opticians are not always well equipped to meet the needs of people with learning disabilities, and so working together to ensure individual needs are accommodated is a vital tool in enhancing care (Pilling 2011).

Hearing difficulties are estimated to affect up to 40 per cent of people with learning disabilities, with causes ranging from structural abnormalities to impacted ear wax. Similar themes are evident in issues around hearing loss to that of sight, with difficulties in the individual communicating problems, and carer awareness or assumptions meaning identification and intervention are often delayed or do not happen (McShae 2014).

Intervention to improve and promote ear and hearing care should also follow the same pattern, with improved awareness and basic care meaning that hearing issues are considered and any changes addressed.

Tests for hearing are by audiologists and can now be accessed in many places where sight tests are administered, meaning that referral from GPs is not now always required. Information and awareness of these services should be made available to people with learning disabilities and their carers, who should again work with the hearing specialists to ensure that individual needs are met.

Another aspect of sensory impairment experienced by a significant number of people with learning disabilities, especially when they may also have autism, is sensory integration, or sensory processing. Difficulties occur when the messages received by the brain from sensory stimuli are not translated effectively into an expected physical response.

Problems can be evident with both under-responsiveness (where a person may not react to sensory stimuli or appear withdrawn), and over-responsiveness (where even very weak stimuli can provoke an exaggerated or extreme response). It is possible for just one, or all, of the senses to be affected, and the five traditional senses of taste, touch, sight, sound and smell; senses controlling movement are also commonly impacted, meaning mobility may be compromised. Changes and fluctuations to a person's sensory processing capacity are often seen and can be as a result of anxiety.

Sensory processing issues can make it hard for individuals to communicate, learn and complete everyday tasks, which could mean difficulties with independent living, relationships or employment. It is important to recognise if someone is experiencing sensory processing difficulties and consider if this could be the reason for behaviour or unusual responses. It may be possible to support people through adaptations to environments, or ways of communicating with individuals, but it might also be necessary to seek additional support from a specialist occupational therapist or other professional with specialist knowledge in this area.

*Implications for practice*

- People with learning disabilities should have regular checks of both hearing and vision, and should be supported to wear corrective appliances if appropriate.
- Sensory issues should be considered as a potential cause of unusual or difficult behaviours, and relevant assessment and investigations should be undertaken.
- Carers should have information on how to perform basic eye and ear care tasks and what to look for and who to go to if they have any concerns about a person's sensory health.
- Accessible information about sensory issues and checks should be provided to increase awareness for people with learning disabilities and those who support them.

**FURTHER READING**

- Hearing and Learning Disability, www.hald.org.uk/.
- Royal National Institute for the Blind (RNIB), www.rnib.org.uk/.
- Seeability. (no date) *Vision and people with learning disabilities: Guidance for GPs* (Seeability).
- Sense, www.sense.org.uk/.
- Sensory Processing Foundation, www.spdfoundation.net/.

## serious case reviews

SEE ALSO **criminal justice; radicalisation; safeguarding**

Over the last decade or so there has been a worrying number of instances of abuse, neglect and even murder of people with learning disabilities in the UK. Many of these cases have involved people who were known to social work, education and healthcare services. Such tragedies require a full investigation into the roles of local professionals and services supporting the individual, whether they be an adult or a child. These investigations may be termed serious case reviews (SCR), case management reviews (CMR) in Northern Ireland, or serious incidents requiring investigation (SIRI).

Children's safeguarding reviews and investigations should be undertaken using a systems approach that adopts a learning stance rather than a blame-seeking approach. However, this is not the same as a 'no-blame' approach nor is it a tolerance for an absence of accountability (SCIE 2012).

When an adult dies as a result of abuse or neglect and there is reason to believe that a partner agency could have worked more effectively to protect the adult, a local authority Safeguarding Adults board must conduct a safeguarding adults review under section 44 of the Care Act 2014.

SCRs have two key functions:

1. Rigorous examination and systematic analysis of the facts.
2. Learning lessons for the future.

Reports emanating from children's and adults' SCRs are presented in an accepted format that includes sections on background, key issues and recommendations.

SCRs have been used to examine failures in safeguarding procedures in individual cases, such as the murders of Steve Hoskin in Cornwall and Ray Atherton in Merseyside, both in 2007. They were both tortured and killed by people who they had previously thought of as friends, but the subsequent reviews found evidence of missed warning signs and failures of communication between police, health and social care services. These reviews, alongside others, led to a greater awareness of what has become recognised as disability hate crime.

SCRs have also exposed institutional failures such as those in Cornwall in 2006, which highlighted widespread financial and physical abuse including using patients' money to fund property improvements and tying patients to their beds for up to 16 hours per day, along with failings in adherence to policy and legislation. Unsurprisingly, the report found that management was poor and that staff training was not prioritised.

The Sutton and Merton enquiry the following year reviewed care provided by Orchard Hill, which was the largest long-stay hospital for people with learning disabilities in the country at that time. The report exposed the rape of a female patient by a male worker and many other incidents of physical, psychological and sexual abuse. Alongside this catalogue of abuse and neglect, there were also reports of lack of staff training, especially in terms of adult protection and risk management. The report highlighted poor management, with a lack of consultation with the patients about their care and treatment leading to a loss of dignity, rights and choice.

These issues have been implicated in the poor care of people with learning disabilities found in other NHS hospitals in subsequent years.

Reviews of private hospitals have also revealed shocking cases of physical and psychological abuse, most recently in the case exposed by BBC television of abuse in a private hospital run by Castlebeck Care in 2011 (*Undercover Care* 2011). The scandal at Winterbourne View prompted the Care Quality Commission (the national regulator) to review care in other hospitals run by Castlebeck, four of which, including Winterbourne View, were subsequently closed. A SCR of these and other cases revealed a pattern of poor management, under-staffing and lack of staff training. This prompted a whole system review of the use of long-stay assessment and treatment facilities, resulting in the publication of the *Transforming Care* (Department of Health 2015b) next-steps review and *Building the Right Support* (Houlden 2015).

Sadly, neglect is not only found in the care of people living with learning disabilities, it also reaches to the care of the deceased. The 2015 review of Southern Health NHS, prompted by the death of Connor Sparrowhawk (also known as 'laughing boy' in the Justice for LB campaign), found that only 1 per cent of premature deaths of people with learning disabilities were investigated in the Oxford hospital.

While such investigations and reports provide evidence from which lessons can be learned about staffing, management and interprofessional working, they can also highlight some of the difficulties experienced by well-trained staff in their work with abusive families.

While a recent systematic review of SCRs confirmed the above themes of poor communication between services, poor management and poor training, perhaps more surprisingly another theme of services failing to protect people with learning disabilities due to intimidation by parents also emerged. In one example, staff appear to have appeased parents and failed to challenge them when they were suspicious of abuse because they feared that parents would stop an individual from attending services, thus depriving them of a safe place (Manthorpe & Martineau 2013).

*Implications for practice*

- SCRs repeatedly highlight themes that in hindsight should have alerted those involved to the potential dangers inherent in a particular case.
- This does not always account for the stress experienced by the worker in a given situation, the guile of the perpetrators of abuse or the organisational context within which day-to-day decisions are made.
- Best practice indicates that professionals need to be well supported by managers and be given time to manage complex cases.
- Information should be sought from and shared between all agencies involved with a case while also working within the parameters of confidentiality.

**FURTHER READING**

- Hull Safeguarding Adults Partnership Board. (2014) *A decade of serious case reviews: A collation of 74 national adult SCRs* (Hull: Safeguarding Adults Partnership Board).
- NSPCC, serious case review information, www.nspcc.org.uk/preventing-abuse/child-protection-system/england/serious-case-reviews/.

## sexuality

SEE ALSO **care planning; discrimination; mental capacity; safeguarding; spirituality**

Sexuality is complex and covers a wide range of human experiences. It is reflected in our values, our sense of self and our self-image and the quality of our relationships. Incorporated into the concept of sexuality are sensuality, intimacy and relationships, gender/sexual identity and sexual health. Each of these components is influenced by an individual's values, culture, experience and spirituality.

The sexual rights of people with learning disabilities have historically been ignored. Often, sexuality only becomes an issue to be discussed when there is a problem. Coping with puberty, sexual identity and sexual feelings can be more difficult for people with learning disabilities who might be struggling to understand their emotions and their body.

The Human Rights Act 1998 enshrines the freedom to express sexuality under article 8, 'Right to respect for private and family life'; article 12, 'Right to marry'; and article 14, 'Prohibition of discrimination'. The White Paper *Valuing People* (Department of Health 2001) states that it is a government objective to enable 'people with learning disabilities to lead full and purposeful lives within their community and to develop a range of friendships, activities and relationships'. *Valuing People* stresses the need for good services to 'help people with learning disabilities develop opportunities to form relationships, including ones of a physical and sexual nature'. *Valuing People Now* (Department of Health 2009a), which improved and developed some of the plans of *Valuing People*, says more about relationships and sexuality and emphasises '...the importance of enabling people with learning disabilities to meet new people, form all kinds of relationships, and to lead a fulfilling life with access to a diverse range of social and leisure activities'. It also highlights 'their right to become parents and the need for adequate support to sustain the family unit' (p. 9).

Despite this guidance and legislation, people with learning disabilities still experience discrimination and poor practice in relation to exploring and developing their sexual identity.

Research has highlighted that for young people with learning disabilities there can still be a number of barriers to expressing their sexuality. There is not a systematic approach to covering sex education within schools, and parents can sometimes struggle with the idea of their child exploring and learning about sexuality. Young people feel that there is a lack of accessible information available to them about sexuality, they want to know about relationships and friendships not just the biological facts, and they also feel that there is a lack of opportunities to meet other young people outside of school or college. Some people from black and minority ethnic (BME) communities are also concerned at a lack of information reflecting their cultural values (University of Leeds Centre for Disability Studies & CHANGE 2009).

The issue of consent is central to discussions around sexuality. The Mental Capacity Act 2005 provides the legislative framework to explore issues of capacity and consent. Given that research (Brown & Turk 1994) suggests that 1400 people with learning disabilities are sexually abused each year, this area cannot be treated lightly. However, it is important that workers fully understand what an assumption of capacity means. There can be a tendency for individual workers and organisations to be risk-averse in this area, and as a result people with learning disabilities can experience restrictions within their lives which are both morally and legally dubious.

Working in the area of sexuality can be challenging. Workers may be asked to address issues which confront or contradict their own value base, and discussions take place in a cultural context where sex and sexuality are often perceived as embarrassing or private, and people with learning disabilities perceived as being either asexual or inappropriately sexual. Workers therefore need to develop an awareness of their own values and judgements, and the way in which they are influenced by the prevailing culture, to ensure that these factors do not impede them in enabling people with learning disabilities to have full access to their rights. Done well, work around sexuality offers people with learning disabilities the opportunity to live full and happy lives and to develop loving and sustaining relationships.

*Implications for practice*

- Person-centred plans and health action plans are key to addressing an individual's wants and needs with regard to sexuality. The plans need to explicitly incorporate sexuality both in its widest context and more specifically.
- Discussions about parenthood are often avoided with people with learning disabilities, as it is frequently seen as potentially problematic. However, in line with the Human Rights Act 1998, it is essential that people with learning disabilities are given the information and support required to make informed decisions about their lives.
- There are a range of resources to support working around sexuality, including booklets, films, teaching packs and CD-ROMs. Some are addressed at people with learning disabilities, some for trainers and some for parents who have children with a learning disability. A comprehensive list can be found in the Appendix of *Talking about sex and relationships* by the University of Leeds Centre for Disability Studies & CHANGE (2009).

**FURTHER READING**

- McCarthy, M. & Thompson, D. (2010) *Sexuality and learning disability* (Pavilion Publishing and Media).
- Barber, C. (2011) Sexuality, relationships and people with a learning disability. *British Journal of Healthcare Assistants,* 5(12), 592–595.

## shared lives

SEE ALSO **accommodation; personalisation**

The Care Quality Commission states that shared lives schemes outperform all other models of care in terms of quality of provision, excelling in the respect and dignity, care and welfare, safeguarding and safety offered to the people who use the schemes (Shared Lives Plus 2015).

Shared lives, originally known as adult placement or family placement, is a model of accommodation and support whereby an adult lives with, or regularly visits, a shared lives carer, effectively living with them as a member of the family. Approximately 7310 people with learning disabilities lived in or used shared life opportunities in England between the years 2013 and 2014 (Shared Lives Plus 2015).

The change of terminology reflects a change in ethos behind the model. At inception, 'adult placement' was developed to mirror the provision of fostering in children's services. The service was originally intended as an alternative to respite care (now more usually termed short breaks), whereby a person with a learning disability would be placed in a local authority (or similar) care unit to enable their family to have a break from caring for them. The change in terminology is more than just semantics – shared lives is about more than simply giving families a break; it is about providing opportunities for adults to experience other ways of living, make new relationships that are valued by them, and broaden their horizons.

Supporters of this model of care celebrate the opportunities that it provides for helping people to enjoy really person-centred support and integration into communities. Shared lives carers often provide opportunities for people with learning disabilities to join in their family activities and become part of their wider social networks. While some people enjoy lifelong commitments and strong relationships with shared life carers, others use the experience as a stepping stone to independence.

Patterns of shared life support differ across the country. In some regions, shared lives carers mainly provide short-term breaks, enabling people to have time away from their families and develop new friendships; other regions tend to adopt a full-time support approach. Shared lives schemes have historically been more popular in the North West of England, although all regions are increasing the numbers of shared lives opportunities as they recognise the opportunities for person-centred care that they provide.

Most shared lives services are provided by third-sector organisations who recruit and provide training and support for the families and individuals who provide the shared life opportunities. Historically most shared lives opportunities have been offered by women or couples, at least one of whom would have had previous experience of either working or caring for a person with a disability in the past. Shared lives providers are not simply altruistic people who 'want to do good', although for some this is an important reason for providing the service. Many report personal gains such as providing company for themselves or their children, giving them an income and getting close to a person with a learning disability for the love that they can bring to a family (McConkey et al. 2005).

*Implications for practice*

- Shared lives is the fastest growing form of care and support in England at the time of writing.

**FURTHER READING**

- Shared Lives Plus. (2015) *The state of shared lives in England*, http://sharedlivesplus.org.uk/images/publications/SL-sector-report-2015.pdf

## siblings

SEE ALSO **parents; loss and grief**

Having a brother or sister with a learning disability can be as rewarding as it is challenging. One study, reported by Contact a Family (2015), suggests that having a sibling with a disability is just like any other sibling relationship except that the feelings are more exaggerated. Feelings including jealousy, love and hate are common in all families and differ from day to day. Siblings often make comparisons between themselves and vie for parental favouritism, so it is crucial that parents try to avoid this, making time to celebrate differences and small achievements of each child. This is the same in any family, whether or not any of the children have disabilities.

**child siblings**

Parents can often feel conflicted when attempting to find a balance of care and support for a child with a disability and a non-disabled sibling. Normal sibling rivalries can be heightened if a child perceives that their sibling is getting more parental attention than they are. So taking time to be with a non-disabled child is crucial to family functioning. Some parents achieve this by building special times into the day, such as bedtime stories, after-school time, weekly outings to the park or other treats to ensure that the non-disabled child can be the centre of parental attention.

Time spent helping a child with a disability to make friendships outside the family unit can pay dividends for families because it helps both siblings to develop individual identities and helps both children to recognise that they do not have to rely solely on their sibling for companionship. Parents may have to spend a little time helping new friends to learn how to interact with a child who has a profound disability or health condition. However, this early experience, that each child is entitled to their own individual life, not dependent upon a brother or sister for care and support and not being expected to be the sole provider of care for a sibling, plays an important role in developing expectations for later in life.

It is important to provide information to child siblings from an early age, especially if their brother or sister has complex needs or a life-limiting condition. In such instances the sibling might need to be told about things that look scary to them such as convulsions or choking. In these cases the siblings should be encouraged to ask questions and have them answered in a matter-of-fact, age-appropriate way, to alleviate potential stress when these things happen.

It might be necessary to prepare a child for the likelihood of their brother or sister needing hospital treatment, which may also require a parent to stay in the hospital with the child. In such instances it may be useful to encourage the sibling to help with packing a bag for the stay, suggesting a favourite cuddly toy that their brother or sister can take with them if appropriate, or perhaps drawing a picture for them or recording a message or playlist to help the hospital room feel more homely.

It is normal at such times for relatives to be worried about the child who is going into hospital, and it is tempting for them to urge the child left at home to 'be good for mummy/daddy'. While this is understandable, it simply puts pressure onto the child and fails to acknowledge their own feelings or fears. It is preferable to ask what they know about the reason for the hospital stay, to listen to their worries and to acknowledge that it must be a difficult time for them too. Relatives and friends who are able to provide treats and distractions for the stay-at-home siblings may be able to help alleviate some of their worries, which in turn helps to support parents.

Most children naturally want to be helpful and to be seen to be caring, so it is unsurprising that they will want to be involved in the care of their sibling. In some cases, children might become young carers helping a parent to manage their sibling's condition. This is particularly common in single-parent families. Brothers and sisters who provide care have rights under the Care Act 2014 (England only), which states that local authorities must consider the young carer's own interests and future endeavours, particularly in areas of study and work, especially for those who are approaching the age of 18.

Sadly, some children will experience the death of their brother or sister. Some might feel responsible for the death, particularly if they had argued or fought shortly before the end or if they feel that they were not supportive enough of their sibling. Some may grieve because they were unable to say goodbye to their sibling in a meaningful way, especially if death occurred in hospital. Reactions of parents will impact greatly on how children experience and deal with these situations. In some instances the parents' own grief may impact on their ability to support their surviving child. Schools should be alert to any changes in behaviour following bereavement and bereaved children may benefit from a referral to Child and Adolescent Mental Health Services.

Sadly, it is common for children who have a disabled sibling to be bullied at school and in the community. Parents should keep the school informed of their child's circumstances, and schools should be vigilant in supporting them. Schools have a responsibility to protect the children in their care and should be able to provide additional support for children in times of distress.

Other support can be found via charitable organisations such as Sibs, which provides lots of useful information for siblings of people with disabilities. Another organisation, Contact a Family, facilitates discussion between families of people with similar conditions. Using these services can help in times of transition and other uncertainties. For example some people find it useful to talk to others who have undergone genetic counselling before deciding whether or not to expose themselves and their children to it.

**adult siblings**

The impact of growing up with a sibling with a disability continues into adult life. Some of this includes feelings and perceived parental expectations of continued care giving, such as providing a home for a sibling. Other issues might include existential feelings within the individual, such as heightened feelings of their own mortality if their sibling died in childhood. In some instances there may be resentment or other difficulties in their relationships with their parents if they perceived them to withdraw love and attention following the death of the other child.

For siblings growing up in happy family homes there can be an expectation of taking on the caring role, including co-residence for their sibling when parents are no longer able to support them in the family home. Families tend to be reluctant to plan for the future of members who have complex disabilities. Reasons for failing to plan include the reluctance of parents to relinquish the caring role, siblings fearing that they are unable or in some cases unwilling to provide levels of care that their parents provided, fear of distressing parents by talking about their decline and eventual death and life stages (e.g. siblings embarking on their own family life), or planning for greater freedom as their own children leave home (Davys, Mitchell & Haigh 2015). Lack of planning can lead to crises if parents die without having discussed the future with their children, including discussions with the child/person with the disability.

Siblings often overestimate the prevalence of disabilities in the general population and may be reluctant to start a family of their own. Those who carry genetic markers for disabilities may worry about reproduction as they develop long-term relationships. This can be particularly problematic while they are deciding whether or not they want to have children of their own. Introducing the topic of reproduction can be tricky for any young couple, and conversations that might include assisted reproduction or adoption can be trickier still. While attitudes towards disabilities have improved over recent years, some couples might find that relatives and friends still hold old-fashioned, prejudicial or oppressive opinions about disability. This can be particularly difficult for couples who may experience pressure from others to terminate a pregnancy that might result in the birth of a baby who has a learning disability.

*Implications for practice*

- Practitioners should be aware of the support needs of siblings. Support might include genetic counselling or help in facilitating conversations in the family.
- Future planning is important for all concerned and needs to be undertaken sensitively.
- It is imperative that the sibling who has the disability is consulted, supported and encouraged to make decisions about their own future at each life stage.
- Siblings are just that, siblings – while some will have a great sense of family togetherness, others will want to move away from their families as soon as possible. This is the same for siblings in families where there is a disability.
- It should not be assumed that the person with the disability wants to continue to live with parents or siblings in later life. Nor should non-disabled siblings feel guilty about wanting to live their own life independent of their brother or sister.

**FURTHER READING**


- Contact A Family, *Siblings*, www.cafamily.org.uk/media/629582/siblings.pdf.
- Sibs, www.sibs.org.uk/.


## spirituality

SEE ALSO **person-centred planning; loss and grief; ethnicity**

Spirituality is the way we find meaning, hope, comfort and inner peace in our life. Many people find spirituality through religion;

others find it through music, art or a connection with nature; and some find it in their values and principles.

Spirituality is concerned with who we are and what life is about. It has to do with our deepest longings; our sadness and joy; our loneliness and friendships; our fears and our times of trust; and our beliefs and disbeliefs. It has to do with the very essence of our being.

Spirituality is part of the core values and ethics of care, and it is expected that professionals will include this aspect of the lives of people with learning disabilities in any care planning and other work they do together. However, some care workers can find it difficult to fully embrace and address spiritual matters with individuals. Some see it as a private matter, or are uncomfortable with it in themselves. Others aren't clear what the term means and may assume it refers only to church-going or other conventional religious activities. In addition, people with learning disabilities are often seen as lacking the capacity for a spiritual life, and can receive a poor welcome in faith communities (Swinton 2002).

Spirituality can be a significant resource which enables people to endure hardship and recuperate from trauma. It can enable people both to emerge from traumatic events more psychologically intact and to recuperate more successfully afterwards (Peres et al. 2007).

Spirituality encompasses a sense of connection with something larger and more enduring than individual identity; the notion of redemption and feelings of love, containment and meaning all contribute to a more robust or resilient psychological infrastructure. It is known that people with learning disabilities are vulnerable to the trauma of abuse, separation, loss and other social and psychological harms as a result of social attitudes to learning disability and the circumstances of prolonged dependency that their disability may require (Brown 2014). Opportunities to develop, strengthen and preserve their spiritual life may therefore be highly significant in enabling people with learning disabilities to survive and thrive.

*Implications for practice*

- Practitioners need to enable people with learning disabilities to discover the best way for them as an individual to experience enthusiasm, inspiration and a sense of connection as part of their day-to-day lives. To do so, practitioners may need to reflect on and overcome their own potential reticence or awkwardness in engaging with spiritual matters.

- As practitioners, we need to view spirituality in its broadest sense and actively, in partnership with people with learning disabilities, seek out opportunities for spiritual growth by assisting in activities such as access to nature, meditation or community singing.

**FURTHER READING**

- Brown, H. (2014) The effectiveness of psychodynamic interventions for people with learning disabilities: a systematic review. *Tizard Learning Disability Review*, *19*(1), 25–28.
- Wilson, C. (2011) Is there a case for community learning disability teams considering the spiritual needs of people with learning disabilities? *Tizard Learning Disability Review*, *16*(3), 31–40.

## syndromes

SEE ALSO **autism; down syndrome; fragile X syndrome; person-centred approaches**

'A syndrome is the medical term for a set of clinical features which commonly occur together' (Mackenzie 2005), and while the majority of learning disabilities have no known cause, there are a number of syndromes that have learning disabilities as a feature.

Syndromes are usually congenital (present at birth) and can result from genetic factors or acquired through issues during pregnancy and birth. In the case of genetic factors, these can be either hereditary (where genes are passed on from parents), as is the case with Fragile X syndrome, or may result from a significant chromosomal abnormality, as would be seen in Patau syndrome where an extra chromosome is present. Acquired syndromes are commonly environmental and most likely result from maternal influences during pregnancy such as illness, diet deficiency or excessive alcohol; for example foetal alcohol syndrome is being increasingly linked to the possible presence of learning disabilities (British Medical Association 2007).

The number of people who would be expected to have a particular syndrome will vary, from Down syndrome which occurs in 1 in every 1000 births (Morris & Alberman 2009), to Rett syndrome where 1 in every 10,000–12,000 births might be expected (NHS Choices 2016b). Others such as Williams syndrome are even less common and may affect only a handful of people.

Where a particular syndrome is suspected by professionals supporting an individual and their families, there may be specific genetic testing that can identify those caused through hereditary means. Where this is the case, parents may be offered advice on the likelihood of the condition occurring in future pregnancies, or within the family, and genetic counselling may be considered. Where causation is not genetic, or there is no specific test, diagnosis may rely on the presence of identified characteristics and a process of differential diagnosis (ruling out other possible causes).

Syndromes may be named after the person who first identified the grouping of features (Prader-Willi syndrome was named after Drs Andrea Prader and Heinrich Willi), or, alternatively, they can refer to one or more of the characteristics of the syndrome (Cri du chat relates to a distinctive high-pitched cry from children with the syndrome that is likened to the cry of a cat – French translation). When the latter is the case, names have come to be seen as negative and devaluing, and in some cases have been changed, for example people with Angelman syndrome (now named after the doctor who described it) used to be referred to as 'puppet children'.

It should be noted that having a specific syndrome does not always mean that the individual will have an accompanying learning disability, and the eventual impact that the condition may have will be determined by not just biological, but also psychological, environmental and social factors.

*Implications for practice*

- It is impossible to know about every syndrome associated with learning disabilities, but when supporting an individual, it may be important to have an understanding of their specific syndrome and its implications for effective intervention.
- Information should be acquired through selection and interpretation of appropriate information from a range of sources, including medical and academic literature as well as from support groups or from other individuals with the syndrome.
- While this research can be done by anyone, professionals such as learning disability nurses and social workers are ideally

placed to carry out this task to inform their own intervention and to present relevant and reliable information to an individual and others.

- Support should take into account any specific needs arising from the syndrome (e.g. health monitoring, behavioural support) but also consider what having the syndrome means for the individual's own personal experience.
- It is important to retain a person-centred approach when supporting an individual with an identified syndrome and not focus solely on the syndrome or the needs arising from it.

**FURTHER READING**


- Gilbert, P. (2000) *A to Z of syndromes and inherited disorders*, 3rd edition (Cheltenham: Nelson Thornes).
- NHS Choices, www.nhs.uk/pages/home.aspx.

# t

## terminology

SEE ALSO **charities and voluntary agencies; legislation; models of disability**

A person who has learning/intellectual disabilities is globally recognised as being a person with an IQ of 70 or less with significant impairment of adaptive functioning (World Health Organization 2007). Internationally, other terms such as developmental delay, mental retardation, mental deficiency and mental handicap are used interchangeably.

This interchangeability can be confusing, particularly in educational settings where 'learning difficulty' is commonly used as an umbrella term to cover conditions such as dyslexia (difficulty in reading); dysgraphia (physical difficulty in forming/writing words); dyspraxia (difficulty with motor skills); or dyscalculia (difficulty with numbers).

The term learning disability is widely recognised in legislation and by support groups across the four countries of the UK. Since the turn of the millennium, there have been calls among some academics and clinicians to adopt the term intellectual disability in response to what many see as the stigmatisation and medicalisation of previous terms (Russell, Mammen & Russell 2005).

In 1996 The World Health Organization (WHO) published the *ICD-10 guide for mental retardation* (World Health Organization 1996) stating that 'retarded' people usually have multiple problems, stemming from an arrested or incomplete development of mind. While noting that the term retardation would be reviewed in ICD-11, the guide went on to describe how different categories of retardation could be initially measured by IQ. Briefly these are *Mild* – IQ of 50–69, *Moderate* – 35–49, *Severe* – 20–34 and *Profound* where the IQ might be estimated to be below 20, this being measured by a person's ability to understand or react to the demands of another person.

Each category is expanded to provide further 'symptoms' to help a clinician make a reasonably accurate diagnosis. Readers will note that while these categories may be useful to clinicians and service developers, they do little to describe the lived experiences of people who are defined under each heading.

By 2010 the definition had been amended, and the once-popular term mental retardation was replaced by intellectual disability. This acknowledged that social upbringing, including poor nutrition and physical health, could also affect cognitive abilities. ICD definitions are qualified by stating that the condition had to be present prior to adulthood. Thus, *acquired brain injury* occurring in adulthood is not considered to be a learning disability.

In the UK, people with learning disabilities prefer to use the term learning disability, eschewing terms such as intellectual disability, special needs and differently abled that the WHO, academics and well-meaning others have used over the last two decades. This is supported by bodies such as the Learning Disability Coalition, which represents 14 individual organisations, as well as the Foundation for People with Learning Disabilities, and the People First movement. Indeed, Bradford People First, a group of people with learning disabilities, successfully campaigned for the removal of the terms 'retard' and 'subnormal' from ICD literature, in favour of learning disabilities.

The outdated terms will be omitted from all WHO publications after 2017, but it is not the only organisation that needs to modernise its terminology. Some services are moving towards a conflation of learning disabilities and learning difficulties, for example LDD (learning difficulties/disabilities) is commonly used in the criminal justice system, and LLDD (learners with learning difficulties and disabilities) or SEN (special educational needs) are preferred in education. Any such changes should be done in consultation and with the agreement of people who have a learning disability.

It may be important for those who plan services and who research illnesses and medical conditions etc. to have agreed terminology; however, it is vital not to insist on academic and clinical terms when working directly with people who may still prefer to use the term learning disability. The right to (re)claim terminology has been acknowledged by other groups, and few would argue with the right of a black person or a gay, lesbian, bisexual or transsexual person to celebrate black or gay pride.

*Implications for practice*

- It may be time to reconsider the perceived pejorative implications of the term learning disability. Respect and meaning can be implied as well as spoken, and it should be acknowledged that many people with learning disabilities have claimed an identity and settled on a term that they can live with.

**FURTHER READING**


- Williams, P. & Evans, M. (2013) *Social work with people with Learning Disabilities*, 3rd edition (London: Learning Matters/Sage).


## transition

SEE ALSO **day services; education; employment; parents of people with learning disabilities**

Transition is a term used in health, social care and educational services to describe the move from children's to adult provision. Typically, it refers to a move from children and family services to adult social care. It may also mean leaving school and moving into further education or work and from paediatric to adult health services.

Above all else, the transition should be undertaken with an understanding that the needs and wishes of the young person should be central to all plans. Person-centred planning using circles of support is essential if the transition is to be experienced as a positive change rather than a maturational necessity.

Transition planning should start when a child reaches school year nine, typically at 13–14 years of age. The child's school has a duty to inform the local authority children and families service prior to the year nine review. This service should assess whether or not the child and their family are likely to need support from adult services during transition, and alert the necessary services where this is indicated. Some local authorities will have specialist transitions workers who will work with a family throughout the process; others may employ two or more workers, typically a children and family social worker and an adult services social worker, perhaps working alongside a learning disability nurse. A Connexions worker should also attend the year nine transition meeting to begin to discuss options such as carrying on to further education or moving into employment. In recent years, adult services eligibility thresholds have meant that many transition meetings have taken place without adult services social workers in attendance. Recent research indicates that lack of involvement in transition meetings by adult services social workers can negatively impact on transition, as fewer options and choices tend to be offered in their absence (Kaehne & Beyer 2014).

In most instances, young people will continue to live at home with their parents when they leave school; however, this might not be the case for all, particularly those children with complex health needs who were educated in residential schools. In such instances it is essential that housing and health representatives attend the year nine review because the young person's health needs might require adaptations to be made to the family home, or they might continue to need specialist residential healthcare. Some individuals might choose to live apart from their families in specialist housing using assistive technologies that enable them to live independently. In such cases, planning can take years, as such housing has to be planned into local authority development plans.

Further complications might occur if the child and their parents live in different local authority areas, especially if the parents have moved away from the local authority that initially assessed the suitability of the out-of-area placement. If a child is dependent on specialist equipment, the transition plan will need to determine ownership of the equipment; for instance it might belong to a residential school or the local health authority. In such cases, the family or the returning local services will have to plan for replacement equipment to be available when the child transitions to adulthood. The purchase of equipment may raise anxieties for parents, particularly those who have been used to equipment being provided free of charge from children's health or social care services. Adult services might subsidise equipment but rarely purchase it outright for individuals.

Funding can be contentious during transition, as it is not only equipment that incurs a cost. Parents who have been used to their son or daughter spending most of their days in school may be dismayed at the prospect of paying for adult daytime support. An area where this is very keenly experienced is in support of children and young people who have life-limiting conditions. In such instances ongoing support might be managed by a carefully negotiated combination of hospice care and direct payments to enable the young person to access community resources when they are feeling well enough.

Transition from childhood to adulthood is a challenging period for most people. For people with learning disabilities and their families, the stage not only signals major changes for the child but also for their parents. School days are generally predictable and parents know when the school term begins and ends. Parents tend to plan their working life around the school day, including taking their child to school or waiting for specialist transport which arrives at predictable times. The transition from full-time education to part-time education, part-time work or enforced idleness can be difficult to adapt to. Families might have developed good relationships with their son or daughter's social worker and school only to have these familiar supports taken away at the same time as their lives change immensely.

During this period, people can experience feelings akin to mourning, sometimes called Transition Shock; this phenomenon has three recognisable stages.

- Stage one – the honeymoon period, the young person and their family look forward to the change, anxiety is tempered by excitement and energy, and they are supported by helpful workers who attempt to make the transition a positive experience.
- Stage two – can be likened to a period of mourning, as people experience the loss of the familiar. The 9am–4pm, five-day-a-week school routine is replaced by maybe two days a week at college, or possibly an individual budget or direct payment that funds a range of activities, which may require negotiations with several workers or organisations who support the young person for 3–4 hours a day for one or more days a week. The young person may mourn the loss of their school friends and teachers and feel isolated. It is important to be aware that this acutely stressful time can lead to some youngsters experiencing a loss of identity and developing mental health problems if the process is

not managed well. They may exhibit changes in their behaviour, becoming angry or withdrawn. Transition plans that take into account hobbies and leisure activities as well as education and employment help militate against these feelings and may enable young people to feel more in control of their lives.

Unfortunately, adult services are generally less well funded than children's services, and adult social workers tend to have larger caseloads than their children and families colleagues, thus making them appear elusive to parents. Parents describe being frustrated by their inability to find someone to help them, often expressing feelings of disappointment and anger. Parents may seek solace in parents' groups and are most likely to complain to social care managers at this time than previously because the support that the family now receives is much less than it was when their son or daughter was a child. Many parents struggle to combine working life with the additional support time that their daughter or son requires. This might lead to loss of income as some parents may have to reduce their working hours or even stop working (Foley et al. 2012).

- Stage three – adjustment. Young people and their families adjust to the new situation, and those who embrace the change may begin to recognise new possibilities. People with learning disabilities are no longer merely expected to waste their days in day centres undertaking menial tasks for a token wage. Creative support can enable a young person to become an entrepreneur, developing their own business or perhaps taking up an internship leading to exciting work possibilities.

*Implications for practice*

- Transition can be a challenging life stage for people with learning disabilities and their parents.
- The key to successful transition is person-centred planning, which takes into account the wishes as well as the needs of the individual. There is some evidence to suggest that transition from school to further education colleges merely delays the eventual transition to employment or other support systems, and that more attention should be paid to preparing people for vocational rather than education-based employment. Alternative community or home-based options might also be considered

as valued alternatives to further education, particularly where people have profound and complex disabilities and may not be able to leave their home often. In such cases, virtual reality experiences have been shown to be effective in helping to increase self-esteem (Weiss, Bialik & Kizony 2003).
- Care must be taken when conducting person-centred transition meetings to ensure that they truly provide a person-centred plan, rather than merely preparing youngsters for service-led provision in a person-centred way (Kaehne & Beyer 2014).

## FURTHER READING

- Preparing for Adulthood, www.preparingforadulthood.org.uk/.
- Transition Information Network, www.transitioninfonetwork.org.uk/.

# references

Action for Advocacy. (2008) *Lost in translation: Towards an outcome focused approach to advocacy provision* (London: Action for Advocacy).

Action for Advocacy. (2011) *Advocacy in a cold climate* (London: Action for Advocacy).

Alzheimer's Society. (2013) *What is dementia* (Factsheet) (London: Alzheimer's Society).

American Psychiatric Association. (2013) *DSM-V Diagnostic and statistical manual of mental disorders*, 5th edition (Arlington, VA: American Psychiatric Association).

Atkinson D. (2004) Research and empowerment: Involving people with learning difficulties in oral and life history research. *Disability & Society, 19*, 691–702.

Autism Act 2009, chapter 15 (London: The Stationery Office).

Azam, K., Sinai, A. & Hassiotis, A. (2009) Mental ill-health in adults with learning disabilities. *Psychiatry, 8*(10), 376–381.

Baird, G., Simonoff, E., Pickles, A., Chandler, S., Loucas, T., Meldrum, D. & Charman, T. (2006) Prevalence of disorders of the autism spectrum in a population cohort of children in South Thames: The Special Needs and Autism Project (SNAP). *Lancet, 368*(9531), 210–215.

Banham Bridges, K.M. (1927) Factors contributing to juvenile delinquency. *Journal of American Institute of Criminal Law and Criminology, 17*(4), 531–580.

Barnes, C. (1992) *An exploration of the principles for media representations of disabled people* (Halifax: The British Council of Organisations of Disabled People and Ryburn Publishing).

Beadle-Brown, J., Richardson, L., Guest, C., Malovic, A., Bradshaw, J. & Himmerich, J. (2014) *Living in fear: Better outcomes for people with learning disabilities and autism*, main research report (Canterbury: Tizard Centre, University of Kent).

Bernard, S. & Turk, J. (2009) *Developing mental health services for children and adolescents with learning disabilities: A toolkit for clinicians* (London: RCPsych Publications).

Bigby, C. (2005) Growing old: Adapting to change and realizing a sense of belonging, continuity and purpose. In G. Grant, P. Goward,

M. Richardson & P. Ramcharan (Eds.), *Learning disabilities: A lifecycle approach to valuing people* (Maidenhead: Open University Press).

Bigby, C., Frawley, P. & Ramcharan, P. (2014) Conceptualizing inclusive research with people with intellectual disability. *Journal of Applied Research in Intellectual Disabilities, 27*, 3–12.

Black, D. (1980) *Inequalities in health: Report of a research working group* (London: Department of Health and Social Security).

BMJ – author not stated. (1904) The care of the epileptic and feebleminded. *British Medical Journal, 2*, 23–24.

Boucher, J. (2009) *The autistic spectrum: Characteristics, causes and practical issues* (London: Sage Publications).

Bradley, H. (2012) Assessing and developing successful communication. In P. Lacey & C. Oyvry (Eds.), *People with profound & multiple disabilities: A collaborative approach to meeting complex needs* (Oxon: Routledge).

Brennan, S. (2013) *Hearing and learning disabilities*, www.ldw.org.uk/media/108420/llais108-hearing.pdf (date accessed 17 February 2016).

*Brilliant Young Mind.* (2014) Directed by Morgan Matthews, Samuel Goldwin Films.

British Institute of Learning Disabilities. (2014) *BILD Code of Practice for minimising the use of restrictive physical interventions: planning, developing and delivering training*, 4th edition (Kidderminster: BILD).

British Medical Association. (2007) *Foetal alcohol spectrum disorders: A guide for healthcare professionals* (BMA: London).

British Psychological Society. (2015) *Dementia and people with intellectual disabilities*, www.bps.org.uk/networks-and-communities/member-microsite/division-clinical-psychology/publications (date accessed 17 November 2015).

Brown, H. (2014) The effectiveness of psychodynamic interventions for people with learning disabilities: A systematic review. *Tizard Learning Disability Review, 19*(1), 25–28.

Brown, H. & Craft, A. (Eds). (1989) *Thinking the unthinkable: Papers on sexual abuse and people with learning difficulties* (London: Family Planning Association Education Unit).

Brown, H. & Smith, H. (1989) Whose 'ordinary life' life is it anyway? *Disability, Handicap and Society, 4*(2), 105–119.

Brown, H. & Turk, V. (1994) Sexual abuse in adulthood: Ongoing risks for people with learning disabilities. *Child Abuse Review, 3*(1), 26–35.

Brownridge, D.A. (2006) Partner violence against women with disabilities. *Violence Against Women, 12*(9), 805–822.

Brugha, T., Cooper, S.A., McManus, S., Purdon, S., Smith, J., Scott, F.J., Spiers, N. & Tyrer, F. (2012) *Estimating the prevalence of autism spectrum conditions in adults: Extending the 2007 adult psychiatric morbidity survey* (London: NHS Information Centre for Health and Social Care).

Bubb, S. (2014) *Winterbourne View – time for change: Transforming the commissioning of services for people with learning disabilities and/or autism* (London: Transforming Care and Commissioning Steering Group).

Bubb, S. (2016) *Time for change: The challenge ahead* (London: ACEVO).

Burke, C. & Ball, K. (2015) *A guide to circles of support* (London: Foundation for People with Learning Disabilities).

Care Act 2014, chapter 23 (London: The Stationery Office).

Carpenter, B. (2000) Sustaining the family: Meeting the needs of families of children with disabilities. *British Journal of Special Education, 27*(3), 135–144.

Chadwick, D. & Jolliffe, J. (2009) A descriptive investigation of dysphagia in adults with intellectual disabilities. *Journal of Intellectual Disability Research, 53*, 29–43.

CHANGE. (2009) *My pregnancy, my choice: A guide to pregnancy in pictures and easy words* (Leeds: CHANGE publications).

CHANGE. (2012) *You and your baby 0–1: Looking after your baby in easy words and pictures* (Leeds: CHANGE publications).

CHANGE. (2013) *You and your little child 1–5: A guide for parents in pictures and easy words* (Leeds: CHANGE publications).

Children Act 1989, chapter 41 (London: The Stationery Office).

Children and Families Act 2014, chapter 6 (London: The Stationery Office).

Children's Learning Disability Nursing Team, Leeds. (2009) *Puberty and sexuality for children and young people with a learning disability: A supporting document for national curriculum objectives* (Leeds: NHS Leeds).

Clark, M.L. (1894) *The relationship of imbecility, pauperism and crime*, https://ia601608.us.archive.org/34/items/ArenaMagazine-Volume10/189406-arena-volume10-x.pdf#page=814&zoom=auto,-13,310 (date accessed 3 March 2016).

Cleaver, H. & Nicholson, D. (2007) *Parental learning disability and children's needs* (Nottingham: DCSF Publications).

Cooper, S. A. & Simpson, M. (2006) Assessment and classification of psychiatric disorders in adults with learning disabilities. *Psychiatry, 5*(9), 306–311.

Contact a Family. (2013) *Fragile X syndrome*, www.cafamily.org.uk/medical-information/conditions/f/fragile-x-syndrome/ (date accessed 15 June 2013).

Contact a Family. (2015) *Siblings: Information for parents of disabled children in England, Northern Ireland, Scotland and Wales* (London: Contact a Family).

Corcoran, H., Lader, P. & Smith, K. (2015) Hate crime: England and Wales 2014/15, Statistical Bulletin 05/15 (London: Home Office).

Council for Disabled Children. (2015) *Every disabled child matters: Right from the start – what we want from the next government* (London: Council for disabled Children).

Criminal Justice Act 2003, chapter 44 (London: The Stationery Office).

Crown Prosecution Service. (2015) *Guidance of prosecuting disability hate crime*, www.cps.gov.uk/legal/d_to_g/disability_hate_crime/ (date accessed 17 December 2015).

Davys, D., Mitchell, D. & Haigh, C. (2015) Futures planning – adult sibling perspectives. *British Journal of Learning Disabilities*, 43, 219–226.

Deacon, J. (1974), *Tongue tied: Subnormality in the seventies* (London: National Society of Mentally Handicapped Children).

Department for Constitutional Affairs. (2007) *Mental Capacity Act 2005 Code of Practice* (London: The Stationery Office).

Department for Education. (2015) *Special educational needs and disability code of practice: 0–25 years* (London: HMSO).

Department for Education. (2016) *Step up to social work: Information for applicants*, www.gov.uk/guidance/step-up-to-social-work-information-for-applicants (date accessed 7 February 2016).

Department for Education and Skills. (2002) *Code of Practice on the education and assessment of special educational needs* (London: HMSO).

Department for Education and Skills (2014) *Special educational needs and disability: Guidance for parents* (London: HMSO).

Department of Health. (1998) *Signposts for Success in commissioning and providing health services for people with learning disabilities* (London: The Stationery Office).

Department of Health. (2000) *Framework for the assessment of children in need and their families* (London: DH).

Department of Health. (2001) *Valuing People: A new strategy for learning disability for the 21st century* (London: DH).

Department of Health. (2004) *National service framework for children, young people and maternity services* (London: DH).

Department of Health (2006) *Our Health, Our Care, Our Say: A new direction for community services* (London: DH).

Department of Health. (2007) *Putting People First: A shared vision and commitment to the transformation of adult social care* (London: DH).

Department of Health. (2008) *End of life care strategy: Promoting high quality care for all adults at the end of life* (London: DH).

Department of Health. (2009a) *Valuing People Now: A new three year strategy for people with learning disabilities* (London: DH).

Department of Health. (2009b) *Valuing Employment Now: Real jobs for people with learning disabilities* (London: DH).

Department of Health. (2010) *Fulfilling and rewarding Lives: The national strategy for adults with autism* (London: DH).
Department of Health. (2011a) *Positive Practice, Positive Outcomes: A handbook for professionals in the criminal justice system working with offenders with learning disabilities* (London: DH).
Department of Health. (2011b) *Staying Positive: The criminal justice system and learning disabilities* (London: DH).
Department of Health. (2012) *Transforming Care: A national response to the Winterbourne View Hospital* (London: DH).
Department of Health. (2014a). *Think Autism: An update to the government adult autism strategy* (London: DH).
Department of Health. (2014b) *Positive and Proactive Care: Reducing the need for restrictive interventions* (London: DH).
Department of Health. (2015a) *Mental Health Act 1983: Code of practice* (London: DH).
Department of Health. (2015b) *Transforming Care for people with learning disabilities – next steps* www.england.nhs.uk/learningdisabilities/care/ (date accessed 19 November 2015).
Department of Health & Department for Education and Skills. (2007) *Good practice guidance on working with parents with a learning disability* (London: DH).
Department of Health & the Home Office. (2000) *No Secrets: guidance on developing and implementing multi-agency policies and procedures to protect vulnerable adults from abuse* (London: DH).
Disability and Discrimination Act 1995, chapter 50 (London: The Stationery Office).
Duffy, S. (2010) The citizenship theory of social justice: Exploring the meaning of personalisation for social workers. *Journal of Social Work Practice, 24*(3), 253–267.
Duffy, S. & Sanderson, H. (2005) Relationship between care management and person centred planning. In P. Cambridge & S. Carnaby (Eds.), *Person centred planning and care management with people with learning disabilities* (London: Jessica Kingsley Publishers).
Duffy, S. & Smith, S. (2007) Person centred partnerships. In J. Thompson, J. Kilbane & H. Sanderson (Eds.), *Person centred practice for professionals* (Maidenhead: Open University Press).
Dunkley, S. & Sales, R. (2014) The challenges of providing palliative care for people with intellectual disabilities: A literature review. *International Journal of Palliative Nursing, 20*(6), 279–284.
Education Act 1981, chapter 60 (London: The Stationery Office).
Education Act 1996, chapter 56 (London: The Stationery Office).

Elementary Education Act 1870.

Emerson, E. (1995) *Challenging behaviour: Analysis and intervention in people with learning disabilities* (Cambridge: Cambridge University Press).

Emerson, E. (2001) *Challenging behaviour: Analysis and intervention in people with learning disabilities*, 2nd edition (Cambridge: Cambridge University Press).

Emerson, E. (2009) *Estimating future numbers of adults with profound multiple learning disabilities in England* (Lancaster: Centre for Disability Research).

Emerson, E. & Baines, S. (2010a) *The estimated prevalence of autism among adults with learning disabilities in England* (London: The Learning Disability Observatory).

Emerson, E. & Baines, S. (2010b) *Health inequalities and people with learning disabilities in the UK: 2010* (Durham: Improving Health & Lives Learning Disabilities Observatory).

Emerson, E. & Baines, S. (2011) Health inequalities and people with learning disabilities in the UK. *Tizard Learning Disability Review, 16*(1), 42–48.

Emerson, E. & Hatton, C. (2007a) Contribution of socioeconomic position to health inequalities of British children and adolescents with Intellectual disabilities. *American Journal of Mental Retardation, 112*, 140–150.

Emerson, E. & Hatton, C. (2007b) *The mental health of children and adolescents with learning disabilities in Britain*, www.lancs.ac.uk/staff/emersone/FASSWeb/Emerson_07_FPLD_MentalHealth.pdf (date accessed 12 December 2015).

Emerson, E., Malam, S., Davies, I. & Spencer, K. (2005) *Adults with learning difficulties in England 2003/4*, www.lancs.ac.uk/staff/emersone/FASSWeb/Emerson_05_ALDE_Main.pdf (date accessed 30 March 2016).

Empowerment Matters CIC & the National Development Team for Inclusion. (2014) *Advocacy charter & code of practice revised edition*, www.qualityadvocacy.org.uk/wp-content/uploads/2014/03/Code-of-Practice.pdf (date accessed 28 February 2016).

Epilepsy Action. (2013) *Vagus nerve stimulation therapy in epilepsy*, www.epilepsy.org.uk/info/treatment/vns-vagus-nerve-stimulation (date accessed 4 February 2016).

Equality Act 2010, chapter 15 (London: The Stationery Office).

Fatimilehin, I.A. & Nadirshaw, Z. (1994) A cross-cultural study of parental attitudes and beliefs about learning disability (mental handicap). *Mental Handicap Research, 7*, 202–227.

Fevre, R., Robinson, A., Lewis, D. & Jones, T. (2013) The ill-treatment of disabled employees in British workplaces. *Work, Employment and Society, 27*(2), 28–37.

Finkelstein, V. (1993) Disability: A social challenge or an administrative responsibility. In J. Swain, V. Finkelstein, S. French & M. Oliver (Eds.), *Disabling barriers – enabling environments* (London: Sage, in association with the Open University).

Florentin, M. (1968) The Sheldon report on child welfare centres: By a Subcommittee of the Standing Medical Advisory Committee of the Minister of Health of the U.K.. *Developmental Medicine & Child Neurology, 10*, 260–261.

Foley, K., Dyke, P., Girdler, S., Bourke, J. & Leonard, H. (2012) Young adults with intellectual disability transitioning from school to post-school: A literature review framed within the ICF. *Disability & Rehabilitation, 34*(20), 1747–1764.

Foundation for People with Learning Disabilities. (2012a) *Learning disability statistics: employment*, www.learningdisabilities.org.uk/help-information/Learning-Disability-Statistics-/187693/ (date accessed 11 November 2015).

Foundation for People with Learning Disabilities. (2012b) *Learning difficulties and ethnicity: Updating a framework for action* (London: Foundation for People with Learning Disabilities).

Foundation for People with Learning Disabilities. (2014a) *Thinking skills programme for people with learning disabilities* (London: Foundation for People with Learning Disabilities).

Foundation for People with Learning Disabilities. (2014b) *We want to be seen and heard* (London: Foundation for People with Learning Disabilities).

Frontline. (2015) *Our programme*, www.thefrontline.org.uk/our-programme (date accessed 7 February 2016).

Fyson, R. & Kitson, D. (2007) Independence or protection – does it have to be a choice? Reflections on the abuse of people with learning disabilities in Cornwall. *Critical Social Policy, 27*(3), 426–436.

Garner, R. (2014) Pupils with special needs are being failed by mainstream schools says mencap. *The Independent*, 14 December 2014, www.independent.co.uk/news/education/education-news/pupils-with-special-needs-are-being-failed-by-mainstream-schools-says-mencap-9923366.html (date accessed 29 July 2016).

Gates, B., Fearns, D. & Welch, J. (2015) *Learning disability nursing at a glance* (Oxford: John Wiley & Sons).

Gayle, D. (2015) Hospital says sorry for do not resuscitate order on man with Down's syndrome. *The Guardian*, 8 December 2015, www.theguardian.com/society/2015/dec/08/hospital-says-sorry-for-do-not-resuscitate-order-on-man-with-downs-syndrome (date accessed 31 January 2016).

GMC. (2016) *Learning disabilities: discrimination*, www.gmc-uk.org/learningdisabilities/200.aspx (date accessed 28 February 2016).

Gore, N.J., McGill, P., Toogood, S., Allen, D., Hughes, J.C., Baker, P., Hastings, R.P., Noone, S.J. & Denne, L.D. (2013) Definition and scope for positive behavioural support. *International Journal of Positive Behavioural Support*, *3*(2), 14–23.

Grundy, D. (2011) Friend or fake? Mate crimes and people with learning disabilities. *Journal of Learning Disabilities and Offending Behaviour*, *2*(4), 167–169.

Guzman, J. (2014) Health beliefs and access to services in an ethnic minority population. *Learning Disability Practice*, *17*(4), 30–33.

Hagerman, R.J. & Hagerman, P.J. (2002) *Fragile x syndrome: Diagnosis, treatment & research*, 3rd edition (Baltimore: John Hopkins University Press).

Harding, C. & Wright, J. (2010) Dysphagia: The challenge of managing eating and drinking difficulties in children and adults who have learning disabilities. *Tizard Learning Disability Review*, *15*(10), 4–14.

Health and Safety Executive. (2015) *Frequently asked questions (what is a hazard? & what is a risk?)*, www.hse.gov.uk/risk/faq.htm (date accessed 31 March 2016).

Health and Social Care Act 2012, chapter 7 (London: The Stationery Office).

Healthcare Careers. (2016) *Learning disability nurse*, www.healthcareers.nhs.uk/explore-roles/nursing/learning-disability-nurse (date accessed 7 February 2016).

Healthier Together. (2014) *A guide to best care Greater Manchester health and social care reform*, https://healthiertogethergm.nhs.uk/resources/consultation-documentation/ (date accessed 20 February 2016).

Heer, K., Larkin, M., Burchess, I. & Rose, J. (2015) The experiences of British South Asian carers caring for a child with developmental disabilities in the UK. *The Tizard Learning Disability Review*, *20*(4), 228–238.

Helen Sanderson Associates. (2015) *One page profiles in healthcare*, www.helensandersonassociates.co.uk (date accessed 31 January 2016).

Helen Sanderson Associates. (2016a) *Communication chart*, www.helensandersonassociates.co.uk/person-centred-practice/person-centred-thinking-tools/communication-chart/ (date accessed 4 February 2016).

Helen Sanderson Associates. (2016b) *Person centred thinking tools*, www.helensandersonassociates.co.uk/person-centred-practice/person-centred-thinking-tools/ (date accessed 16 February 2016).

Helen Sanderson Associates. (2016c) *Matching support*, www.helensandersonassociates.co.uk/person-centred-practice/person-centred-thinking-tools/matching-support/ (date accessed 16 February 2016).

Hervie, V.M. (2013) *Shut up! Social inclusion of children with intellectual disabilities in Ghana: An empirical study of how parents and teachers experience social inclusion of children with intellectual disabilities*, http://brage.bibsys.no/xmlui/handle/11250/139975 (date accessed 20 November 2015).

Heslop, P., Blair, P., Fleming, P., Hoghton, M., Marriott, A. & Russ, L. (2013) *Confidential inquiry into premature deaths of people with learning disabilities (CIPOLD): Final report* (Bristol: Norah Fry Research Centre).

HM Government. (2011) *Prevent strategy* (London: Crown Copyright).

HM Government. (2015a) *Channel duty guidance: Protecting vulnerable people from being drawn into terrorism – statutory guidance for channel panel members and partners of local panels* (London: Crown Copyright).

HM Government. (2015b) *Working together to safeguard children: A guide to inter-agency working to safeguard and promote the welfare of children* (London: Crown Copyright).

HM Inspectorate of Probation, HMI Constabulary, HM Crown Prosecution Inspectorate & the Care Quality Commission. (2014) *A joint inspection of the treatment of offenders with learning disabilities within the criminal justice system – phase 1 from arrest to sentence* (London: HM Inspectorate of Probation).

Home Office. (2004) *Working within the sexual offences act 2003* (London: Home Office Communications Department).

Houlden, A. (2015) *Building the right support: A national plan to develop community services and close inpatient facilities for people with a learning disability and/or autism who display behaviour that challenges, including those with a mental health condition* (London: Local Government Association; Association of Directors of Adult Social Services; NHS England).

Human Rights Act 1998, chapter 42 (London: The Stationery Office).

Iacono, T., Bigby, C., Carling-Jenkins, R. & Torr, J. (2014) Taking each day as it comes: Staff experiences of supporting people with Down syndrome and Alzheimer's disease in group homes. *Journal of Intellectual Disability Research, 58*(6), 521–533.

In Control. (2014) *History of 'In Control'*, www.in-control.org.uk/about-us/history-of-in-control.aspx (date accessed 19 January 2016).

Jaber, L., Halpem, G.J. & Shohat, T. (2000) Trends in the frequencies of consanguineous marriages in the Israeli Arab community. *Clinical Genetics, 58*, 106–110.

Jackson, M.J. & Turkington, D. (2005) Depression and anxiety in epilepsy. *Journal of Neurology, Neurosurgery & Psychiatry, 76*(supp 1), i45–i47.

Jacoby, A., Gorry, J. & Baker, G.A. (2005) Employers' attitudes to employment of people with epilepsy: Still the same old story? *Epilepsia, 46*(12), 1978–1987.

Johnson, K., Walmsley, J. & Wolfe, M. (2010) *People with intellectual disabilities: Towards a good life* (Bristol: The Policy Press).

Joint Committee on Human Rights. (2008) *A life like any other?: Human rights of adults with learning disabilities,* Seventh report of sessions 2007-8 volume 1 Report and formal minutes (London: House of Lords & House of Commons Joint committee on Human Rights March 2008).

Joint Epilepsy Council of the UK and Ireland. (2011) *Epilepsy prevalence, incidence and other statistics* (Leeds: The Joint Epilepsy Council of the UK and Ireland).

Jones, J. (2002) *BILD factsheet: Communication* (Birmingham: BILD).

Kaehne, A. & Beyer, S. (2014) Person-centred reviews as a mechanism for planning the post-school transition of young people with intellectual disability. *Journal of Intellectual Disability Research, 58*(7), 603–613.

Kaplan, S.G. & Wheeler, E.G. (1983) Survival skills for working with potentially violent clients. *Social Casework: The Journal of Contemporary Social Work, 64*(6), 339–346.

Lawton, A. (2009) *Personalisation and learning disabilities: A review of evidence on advocacy and its practice for people with learning disabilities and high support needs,* Report 24 (London: Social Care Institute for Excellence).

Long, L.A., Roche, J. & Stringer, D. (2010) *The law and social work,* 2nd edition (London: Palgrave Macmillan).

Lord Bradley. (2009) *The Bradley report: Lord Bradley's review of people with mental health problems or learning disabilities in the criminal justice system,* http://webarchive.nationalarchives.gov.uk/20130107105354/www.dh.gov.uk/prod_consum_dh/groups/dh_digitalassets/documents/digitalasset/dh_098698.pdf (date accessed 12 December 2015).

Loucks, N. (2007) *Prisoners with learning difficulties and learning disabilities: Review of prevalence and associated needs* (London: Prison Reform Trust).

Lunedei, E. (1995) Brave Man (Nashville: Arista Records).

*MacIntyre Undercover.* (1999) BBC1, 16 November, 21:00.

Mackenzie, F. (2005) The roots of biomedical diagnosis. In G. Grant, P. Goward, M. Richardson, & P. Ramcharan (Eds.), *Learning disability: A life cycle approach to valuing people* (Maidenhead: Open University Press).

Mansell, J. (1993) *Services for people with learning disabilities and challenging behaviour or mental health needs* (London: DH).

Mansell, J. (2007) *Services for people with learning disabilities and challenging behaviour or mental health needs,* revised edition (London: DH).

Mansell, J. (2010) Raising our sights: services for adults with profound intellectual and multiple disabilities. *Tizard Learning Disability Review*, 15(3), 5–12.

Manthorpe, J. & Martineau, S. (2013) What can and cannot be learned from serious case reviews of the care and treatment of adults with learning disabilities in England? Messages for social workers. *British Journal of Social Work*, 45(1), 331–348.

Marks, D. (1999) *Disability: Controversial debates and psychosocial perspectives* (Routledge: London).

Matthews, D., Gibson, L. & Regnard, C. (2010) One size fits all? Palliative care for people with learning disabilities. *British Journal of Hospital Medicine*, 71(1), 40–43.

Mathews, I. & Crawford, K. (2011) *Evidence-based practice in social work* (Exeter: Learning Matters).

Mazars. (2015) *Independent review of deaths of people with a learning disability or mental health problem in contact with southern health NHS foundation trust April 2011 to March 2015* (London: Mazars LLP).

McConkey, R., McConaghie, J., Roberts, P. & King, D. (2005) Characteristics of people providing family placements to adult persons with intellectual disabilities. *British Journal of Learning Disabilities*, 33, 132–137.

McKenzie, K. & Paxton, D. (2005) *Learning disability screening questionnaire (LDAQ)* (Edinburgh: GCM Records).

McShae, L. (2014) Hearing loss in people with learning disabilities. *British Journal of Healthcare Assistants*, 9(3), 124–127.

Mencap. (2002) *The housing timebomb: The housing crisis facing people with a learning disability and their older parents* (London: Mencap).

Mencap. (2007) *Death by indifference* (London: Mencap).

Mencap. (2012a) *Stuck at home: The impact of day service cuts on people with a learning v disability* (London: Mencap).

Mencap. (2012b) *Death by indifference: 74 deaths and counting* (London: Mencap).

Mencap. (no date) *Postural care: Protecting and restoring body shape* (London: Mencap).

Mental Capacity Act 2005, chapter 9 (London: The Stationery Office).

Mental Capacity Act Deprivation of Liberty Safeguards 2009 (London: The Stationery Office).

Mental Health Act 1983, chapter 20 (London: The Stationery Office).

Mental Health Act 2007, chapter 12 (London: The Stationery Office).

Mental Health Foundation. (2007) *The fundamental facts: The latest facts and figures on mental health* (London: Mental Health Foundation).

Mental Health Research Network – Clinical Research Group Forensic Intellectual and Developmental Disabilities. (2015) *Home page*, www.forensiclearningdisability.com/ (date accessed 12 December 2015).

Michael, J. (2008) *Healthcare for all: Report of the independent inquiry into access to healthcare for people with learning disabilities* (London: Aldrick Press).

Ministry of Justice. (2008a) *Mental Capacity Act 2005: Deprivation of liberty safeguards – Code of Practice to supplement the main Mental Capacity Act 2005 Code of Practice* (London: The Stationery Office).

Ministry of Justice. (2008b) *Thinking skills programme* (London: Crown Copyright).

Mir, G., Tovey, P., Ahmad, W. (2001) *Cerebral palsy and South Asian Communities* (Leeds: Centre for Research in Primary Care – University of Leeds).

Morrell, M.J. (2002) Stigma and epilepsy. *Epilepsy and Behaviour, 3*, S21–S25.

Morris, J.K. & Alberman, E. (2009) Trends in Down's syndrome live births and antenatal diagnoses in England and Wales from 1989 to 2008: Analysis of data from the National Down Syndrome Cytogenetic Register. *British Medical Journal, 339*, b3794.

Moss, S., Prosser, H., Costello, H., Simpson, N., Patel, P., Rowe, S., Turner, S. & Hatton C. (1998) Reliability and validity of the PAS ADD checklist for detecting psychiatric disorders in adults with intellectual disability. *Journal of Intellectual Disability Research, 42*, 173–183.

Murray, M. & Osbourne, C. (2009) *Safeguarding disabled children: Practice guidance* (Nottingham: DCSF Publications).

National Careers Service. (2016) *Job profiles: Special educational needs teacher*, https://nationalcareersservice.direct.gov.uk/advice/planning/job profiles/Pages/SpecialEducationalNeedsTeacher.aspx (date accessed 7 February 2016).

National Health Service and Community Care Act 1990, chapter 19 (London: The Stationery Office).

National Institute for Health and Clinical Excellence. (2010) *Dementia quality standard*, Quality Standard 1 (London: NICE).

National Institute for Health and Clinical Excellence. (2012) *The epilepsies: The diagnosis and management of the epilepsies in adults and children in primary and secondary care*, Clinical Guideline 137 (London: NICE).

National Institute for Health and Clinical Excellence. (2015) *Challenging behaviour and learning disabilities: Prevention and interventions for people with learning disabilities whose behaviour challenges*, Clinical Guideline NG11 (London: NICE).

National Offender Management Service. (2013) *Improving services for offenders with learning disabilities and difficulties* (London: National Offender Management Service).

Neill, M. & Sanderson, H. (2012) *Circles of support and personalisation*, http://community-circles.co.uk/circles-of-support-and-personalisation/ (date accessed 16 February 2016).

NHS Choices. (2014) *Autism and Asperger syndrome: Causes*, www.nhs.uk/Conditions/Autistic-spectrum-disorder/Pages/Causes.aspx (date accessed 2 February 2014).

NHS Choices. (2016a) *Dysphagia (swallowing problems)*, www.nhs.uk/conditions/Dysphagia/Pages/definition.aspx (date accessed 31 March 2016).

NHS Choices. (2016b) *Rett Syndrome*, www.nhs.uk/conditions/rett-syndrome/Pages/Introduction.aspx (date accessed 14 November 2015).

NHS Confederation. (2015) *Joining up health and social care personal budgets: Key points on implementation*, NHS confederation briefing, January 2015, Issue 280.

NHS England. (2015) *Accessible information standard* (Leeds: NHS England).

Nirje, B. (1969) The normalisation principle and its human management implications. Reproduced in *SRV-VRS: The International Social Role Valorisation Journal*, 1(2), 19–23.

Nursing and Midwifery Council. (2016) *Our role*, www.nmc.org.uk/about-us/our-role/ (date accessed 4 December 2015).

O'Brien, J. & Lyle, C. (1987) *A framework for accomplishments: A workshop for people developing better services* (Decatur, GA: Responsive System Associates).

O'Brien, J. & O'Brien, C.L. (2002) The origins of person centred planning: a community practice perspective In S. Holburn & P. Vietze (Eds.), *Person centred planning: Research, practice and future directions* (Baltimore: Paul Brookes Publishing).

O'Brien, J., Pearpoint, J. & Kahn, L. (2010) *The PATH & MAPS handbook: Person centred ways to build community* (Toronto: Inclusion Press).

Ofcom. (2005) *The representation and portrayal of people with disabilities on analogue and terrestrial television: Content analysis research report* (London: Ofcom).

O'Hara, J. (2003) Learning disabilities and ethnicity: Achieving cultural competence. *Advances in Psychiatric Treatment*, 9(3), 166–174.

Oliver, M. (1990) *The individual and social models of disability*, http://disability-studies.leeds.ac.uk/files/library/Oliver-in-soc-dis.pdf (date accessed 12 February 2016).

Oliver, M.J. (1999) Capitalism, disability and ideology: A materialist critique of the normalisation principle. In R. Flynn & A. Lemay (Eds.), *A quarter-century of normalisation and social role valorisation: Evolution and impact* (Ottawa: University of Ottawa Press).

Oliver, M. & Barnes, C. (2006) *Disability politics and the disability movement in Britain: Where did it all go wrong?*, http://disability-studies.leeds.ac.uk/files/library/Barnes-Coalition-disability-politics-paper.pdf (date accessed 5 November 2015).

Olsen, A. & Carter, C. (2016) Responding to the needs of people with learning disabilities who have been raped: Co-production in action. *Tizard Learning Disability Review, 21*(1), 30–38.

Organisation of the Islamic Conference (OIC). (1990) *The Cairo declaration on human rights in Islam*, www.oic-oci.org/english/article/human.htm (date accessed 1 April 2016).

Parr, J.R., Joleff, N., Gray, L., Gibbs, J., Williams, J. & McConachie, H. (2013) Twenty years of research shows UK child development team provision still varies widely for children with disability. *Child: Care, Health and Development, 39*(6), 903–907.

Penny, C. & Exworthy, T. (2015) A gilded cage is still a cage: Cheshire West widens 'deprivation of liberty'. *The British Journal of Psychiatry, 206*(2), 91–92.

Peres, J., Moreira-Almeida, A., Nasello, A. & Koenig, H. (2007) Spirituality and resilience in trauma victims. *Journal of Religion and Health, 46*(3), 343–350.

Pilling, R. (2011) *The management of visual problems in adult patients who have learning disabilities* (London: The Royal College of Ophthalmologists).

Pollard, K., Sellman, D. & Thomas, J. (2014) The need for interprofessional working. In J. Thomas, K. Pollard, & D. Sellman (Eds.), *Interprofessional working in health and social care: Professional perspectives*, 2nd edition (Basingstoke: Palgrave Macmillan).

Porter, E., Kidd, G., Murray, N., Uytman, C., Spink, A. & Anderson, B. (2012) Developing the pregnancy support pack for people who have a learning disability. *British Journal of Learning Disabilities, 40*, 310–317.

Prime Minister's Strategy Unit. (2005) *Improving the life chances of disabled people: A joint report with the Department of Work and Pensions, Department of Health, Department for Education and Skills, Office of the Deputy Prime Minister* (London: Cabinet Office).

Powers, L.E., Curry, M.A., McNeff, E., Saxton, M., Powers, J. & Oschwald, M.M. (2008) End the silence: A survey of the abuse experiences of men with disabilities. *Journal of Rehabilitation, 7*(4), 41–53.

Prospects. (2016) *Job profiles: Social worker*, www.prospects.ac.uk/job-profiles/social-worker (date accessed 7 February 2016).

Public Health England. (2014) *People with learning disabilities in England 2013* (London: Public Health England).

Public Health England. (2015a) *Joint health and social care self assessment framework 2014 – results,* www.improvinghealthandlives.org.uk/projects/jhscsaf2014results (date accessed 31 January 2016).

Public Health England. (2015b) *Reasonable adjustments,* www.improvinghealthandlives.org.uk/projects/reasonableadjustments (date accessed 31 January 2016).

Public Interest and Disclosure Act 1998, chapter 23 (London: The Stationery Office).

*P v Cheshire West and Chester Council* and *P and Q v Surrey County Council,* Supreme Court Judgment, 19 March 2014.

Race, D. (2007) *Intellectual disability: Social approaches* (Berkshire: Open University Press).

Raghavan, R., Marshall, M., Lockwood, A. & Duggan, L. (2004) Assessing the needs of people with learning disabilities and mental illness: Development of the learning disability version of the cardinal needs schedule. *Journal of Intellectual Disability Research, 48*(1), 25–36.

*Rain Man.* (1988) Directed by Barry Levinson, United Artists.

Raphael Leff, J. (1991) *Psychological processes of childbearing* (London: Chapman & Hall).

Reddington, T. & Fitzsimons, J. (2013) People with learning disabilities and microenterprise. *Tizard Learning Disability Review, 18*(3), 124–131.

Rethink Mental Illness. (2015) *Factsheet: Care programme approach* (London: Rethink Mental Illness).

Robertson, J., Hatton, C., Emerson, E. & Baines, S. (2014) The impact of health checks for people with intellectual disabilities: An updated systematic review of evidence. *Research in Developmental Disabilities, 35,* 2450–2462.

Robertson, J., Hatton, C., Emerson, E. & Baines, S. (2015) Prevalence of epilepsy among people with intellectual disabilities: A systematic review. *Seizure: European Journal of Epilepsy, 29,* 46–62.

Roper, N., Logan, W.W. & Tierney, A.J. (2000) *The Roper-Logan-Tierney model of nursing: Based on activities of living* (Edinburgh: Elsevier Health Sciences).

Rose, N., Kent, S. & Rose, J. (2011) Health professionals' attitudes and emotions towards working with adults with intellectual disability (ID) and mental ill health. *Journal of Intellectual Disability Research, 56*(9), 854–864.

Royal College of Psychiatrists. (2013) *People with learning disability and mental health, behavioural or forensic problems: the role of in-patient services* (London: Royal College of Psychiatrists).

Royal National Institute for the Blind. (2016) *Across the spectrum: learning disability and sight loss*, www.rnib.org.uk/services-we-offer-advice-professionals-nb-magazine-health-professionals-nb-features/across-spectrum (date accessed 17 February 2016).

Russell, S., Mammen, P. & Russell, P.S.S. (2005) Emerging trends in accepting the term intellectual disability in the world disability literature. *Journal of Intellectual Disabilities*, 9(3), 187–192.

Ryan, K., McEvoy, J., Guerin, S. & Dodd, P. (2010) An exploration of the experience, confidence and attitudes of staff to the provision of palliative care to people with learning disabilities. *Palliative Medicine*, 24(6), 566–572.

Safeguarding Vulnerable Groups Act 2006, chapter 47 (London: The Stationery Office).

Saha, S., Doran, E., Osann, K.E., Hom, C., Movsesyan, N., Rosa, D.D., Tournay, A. & Lott, I.T. (2014) Self-concept in children with Down syndrome. *American Journal of Medical Genetics, Part A*, 9999, pp. 1–8.

Sanderson, H., Kennedy, J., Ritchie, P., Goodwin, G. (1997) *People, plans & possibilities: Exploring person centred planning* (Edinburgh: SHS Trust).

Sanderson, H. & Lepkowsky, M.B. (2014) *Person centred teams: A practical guide to delivering personalisation through effective team-work* (London: Jessica Kingsley Publishers).

SCIE. (2012) *At a glance 01: Learning together to safeguard children: A 'systems' model for case reviews*, www.scie.org.uk/publications/ataglance/ataglance01.asp (date accessed 14 October 2015).

SCIE. (2015a) *Practice Guide 51: Co-production in social care: What is it and how to do it*, www.scie.org.uk/publications/guides/guide51/ (date accessed 12 April 2016).

SCIE. (2015b) *Practice Guide 37: Good Practice in Social Care for Refugees and asylum seekers*, http://disability-studies.leeds.ac.uk/files/library/Barnes-Coalition-disability-politics-paper.pdf (date accessed 14 December 2015).

Seeability. (no date) *Vision and people with learning disabilities: Guidance for GPs* (Epsom: Seeability).

Sexual Offences Act 2003, chapter 42 (London: The Stationery Office).

Shakespeare, T. & Watson, N. (2001) The social model of disability: An outdated ideology? *Research in social science and disability*, 2, 9–28.

Shared Lives Plus. (2015) *The state of shared lives in England* (Liverpool: Shared Lives Plus).

Sheehan, R., Hassiotis, A., Walters, K., Osborn, D., Strydom, A. & Horsfall, L. (2015) Mental illness, challenging behaviour, and psychotropic drug prescribing in people with intellectual disability: UK population based cohort study. *British Medical Journal*, 351, h4326.

*Silent Minority*. (1981) ITV, 10 June, 21:00.

Sinason, V. (2012) Mental handicap and the human condition: An analytic approach to intellectual disability. *American Journal of Psychoanalysis, 72*(1), 84–86.

Skills for Care. (2014) *A Positive and proactive workforce: A guide to workforce development for commissioners and employers seeking to minimise the use of restrictive practices in social care and health* (Leeds: Skills for Care).

Slevin, E. (2007) Challenging behaviour. In B Gates (Ed.), *Learning disabilities: Towards inclusion* (London: Churchill Livingstone).

Smale, G., Tuson, G., Biehal, N. & Marsh, P. (1993) *Empowerment, assessment, care management and the skilled worker* (London: HMSO).

Special Educational Needs and Disabilities Act 2001, chapter 10 (London: The Stationery Office).

Sutton, C. (2006) *Helping families with troubled children: A preventive approach*, 2nd edition (Chichester: Wiley-Blackwell).

Swinton, J. (2002) Spirituality and the lives of people with learning disabilities. *Tizard Learning Disability Review, 7*(4), 29–35.

Tafirei, P., Makaye, J. & Mapetere, K. (2013) Inclusion and the world of disability: A case study of Zaka central cluster, Masvingo, Zimbabwe. *Journal of African Studies and Development, 5*(8), 241–249.

Talbot, J. (2008) *Prisoner's voices: Experiences of the criminal justice system by prisoners with learning disabilities and difficulties* (London: Prison Reform Trust).

Talbot, J. (2012) *Fair Access to Justice? Support for vulnerable defendants in the criminal justice system* (London: Prison Reform Trust).

*The Girl with the Dragon Tattoo*. (2011) Directed by David Fincher, Columbia Pictures.

The Scottish Government. (2012) *Strengthening the commitment: The report of the UK modernising learning disability nursing review* (Edinburgh: The Scottish Government).

Thompson, D. (2007) Older people with learning disabilities. In B. Gates (Ed.), *Learning Disabilities Toward Inclusion*, 5th edition (Philadelphia: Elsevier).

TLAP. (2016) *What is think local act personal?*, www.thinklocalactpersonal.org.uk/About_us/ (date accessed 19 January 2016).

Tope, R. & Thomas, E. (2007) *Health and social care policy and the interprofessional agenda*, http://caipe.org.uk/silo/files/cipw-policy.pdf (date accessed 20 February 2016).

Towers, C. (2013) *Thinking ahead: Improving support for people with learning disabilities and their families to plan for the future* (London: Foundation of People with Learning Disability).

Tredgold, A.F. (1909) The feebleminded: A social danger. *Eugenics Review, 1*, 97–104.

Turk, J. (2008) *The health and social aspects of fragile x syndrome*, www.fragilex.org.uk (date accessed 15 May 2013).

Turner, S. (2011) Increasing health checks for people with learning disabilities. *Nursing Standard, 36*(7), 35–38.

Turner, S., Giraud-Saunders, A. & Marriott, A. (2013) *Improving the uptake of screening services by people with learning disabilities across the south west peninsula: A strategy and toolkit* (Bath: National Development Team for Inclusion).

*Undercover Care: The abuse exposed.* (2011) BBC1, 31 May, 21:00.

UNESCO (1994) *The Salamanca statement on principles, policy and practice in special needs education*, Paris, France, www.unescobkk.org/education/inclusive-education/what-is-inclusive-education/background/ (date accessed 5 November 2015).

United Nations. (2006) *Convention on the rights of persons with disabilities*, Treaty Series 2515: 3. Print.

United Nations Refugee Agency. (2010) *Convention and protocol relating to the status of refugees* (Geneva: United Nations High Commissioner for Refugees).

University of Leeds Centre for Disability Studies & CHANGE. (2009) *Talking about sex and relationships: The views of young people with learning disabilities* (Leeds: CHANGE publications).

Valuing People Support Team. (2004) *Learning difficulties and ethnicity: A framework for action* (London: DH).

Vanhala, L. (2011) *Making rights a reality? Disability rights activists and legal mobilization* (New York: Cambridge University Press).

Walmsley, J. (2001) Normalisation, emancipatory research and inclusive research in learning disability. *Disability & Society, 16*, 187–205.

Ward, C. (2012) *Perspectives on ageing with a learning disability* (York: Joseph Rowntree Foundation).

Ward, L. (2002) Women with learning disabilities and the menopause. *Tizard Learning Disability Review, 7*(1), 13–16.

Ward, L. & Tarleton, B. (2007) Sinking or swimming? Supporting parents with learning disabilities and their children. *Tizard Learning Disability Review, 12*(2), 22–32.

Waterlow, J. (2005) *The Waterlow pressure ulcer prevention manual* (Wound Care Society).

Weiss, P., Bialik, P. & Kizony, R. (2003) Virtual reality provides leisure time opportunities for young adults with physical and intellectual disabilities. *Cyber Psychology & Behaviour, 6*, 335–342.

Wendell, S. (1989) Towards a feminist theory of disability. In L. J. Davis (Ed.), (2006) *The disability studies reader* (Chicago: Routledge).

Wertheimer, A. (Ed.). (2002) *Today and tomorrow: The report of the growing older with learning disabilities programme* (London: Mental Health Foundation).

Williams, D. (1996) *Autism: An inside out approach* (London: Jessica Kingsley Publishers).

Williams, P. (2009) *Social work with people with learning difficulties* (Exeter: Learning Matters).

Willis, D.S., Wishart, J.G. & Muir, W.J. (2010) Carer knowledge and experiences with menopause in women with intellectual disabilities. *Journal of Policy and Practice in Intellectual Disabilities*, 7(1), 42–48.

Wing, L. (1981) Asperger's syndrome: A clinical account. *Psychological Medicine*, *11*(1): 115–129.

Wing, L. & Gould, J. (1979) Severe impairments of social interaction and associated abnormalities in children: Epidemiology and classification. *Journal of Autism and Childhood Schizophrenia*, 9, 11–29.

Wolfensberger, W. (1972) *The principle of normalisation in human services* (Toronto: National Institute on Mental Retardation).

Wolfensberger, W. (1998) *A brief introduction to social role valorisation as a high-order concept for addressing the plight of socially devalued people and for structuring human services*, 3rd edition (Syracuse: Syracuse University).

Wolfensberger, W., Thomas, S. & Caruso, G. (1996) Some of the 'universal good things in life' which the implementation of social role valorisation can be expected to make more accessible to devalued people. *The International Social Role Valorisation Journal*, 2(2), 12–14.

Wood, L. (2012) *Media representation of disabled people*, www.disabilityplanet.co.uk/critical-analysis.html (date accessed 2 February 2016).

World Health Organization. (1992) *ICD-10 Classification of mental and behavioural disorders: Clinical descriptions and diagnostic guidelines* (Geneva: World Health Organization).

World Health Organization. (1996) *ICD-10 Guide for mental retardation* (Geneva: World Health Organization).

World Health Organization. (2007) *Atlas global resources for persons with intellectual disabilities (Atlas-ID)* (Geneva: WHO Press).

World Health Organization. (2014) *Mental health: Strengthening our response*, www.who.int/mediacentre/factsheets/fs220/en/ (date accessed 14 December 2015).

Young, H., Garrard, B., Lambe, L. & Hogg, S. (2014) Helping people cope with bereavement. *Learning Disability Practice*, 17(6), 16–20.

# index